NARCISSISM AND THE
RELATIONAL WORLD

William G. Herron

University Press of America,® Inc.
Lanham • New York • Oxford

Copyright © 1999 by
University Press of America,® Inc.
4720 Boston Way
Lanham, Maryland 20706

12 Hid's Copse Rd.
Cumnor Hill, Oxford OX2 9JJ

Library of Congress Cataloging-in-Publication Data

Herron, William G.
Narcissism and the relational world / William G. Herron.
p.   cm.
Includes bibliographical references and index.
1. Narcissism. 2. Interpersonal relations. 3. Psychoanalysis. I. Title.
RC553.N36H47   1999   616.85'85—dc21   99—41511 CIP

ISBN 0-7618-1496-5 (cloth: alk. ppr.)
ISBN 0-7618-1497-3 (pbk: alk. ppr.)

⊖™ The paper used in this publication meets the minimum
requirements of American National Standard for Information
Sciences—Permanence of Paper for Printed Library Materials,
ANSI Z39.48—1984

CONTENTS

Preface

This book is a revisionist's view of narcissism. It reflects a major contemporary trend in psychoanalysis, namely an emphasis on subjectivity. Thus far that trend has emphasized the recognition and use of the analyst's subjectivity. Preceding this emphasis it was customary to view the patient as the subject, in fact, so much so that earlier formulations of psychoanalysis have been described as representing a "one-person" psychology. Current psychoanalytic theory and practice are instead depicted as indicative of a "two-person"" psychology. This is based on now moving from an awareness of the inevitability of the analyst's subjectivity, and the corresponding relativity of apparent objectivity, to a focus on intersubjectivity. The analytic process now involves the dialogic or dialectic interaction of two minds, the mind of the analyst and the mind of the patient. On this basis, most if not all psychoanalytic concepts require a new look.

I have chosen narcissism for that purpose because of my previous work in that area, because of the continual interest in narcissistic disorders, and primarily because I believe that narcissism is a particularly useful concept for understanding both subjectivity and intersubjectivity. My thesis is that narcissism is an organizing principle for behavior, in essence a major motivational force that can be healthy or pathological and that illuminates the intricacies of subjectivity for both therapists and patients.

Chapter I establishes the meaning of narcissism, a Janus-like concept from its inception that continues to have that flavor. The definition of narcissism is traced from Freud through ego psychology, relational theorists, and other reformulations. In following this evolution of definitions I have also elaborated on the shift in psychoanalysis from an emphasis on structural theory to relational theory, an elaboration that continues throughout the book. The chapter concludes with a recognition of the lack of a consensus for defining narcissism, but with agreement that it is a particularly important concept. I define it as a personal perspective that operates as a motivational force within a developmental process that can be depicted using the major psychodynamic conceptions of psychoanalysis.

Chapter II is concerned with narcissism in developmental processes, beginning with the concept of the self. This is also a difficult construct to define, but its existence is generally agreed upon, as well as the importance of subjective experience and subjective states in relation to others. The developmental progression of narcissism as a personal perspective is then described. The direction of narcissism is depicted within major developmental schema such as psychosexual, relational, and self. Such consideration leads to an overview of the major theorists of pathological narcissism. Although there are definitely different types of narcissistic pathology, and a variety of etiologies proposed, the latter tend to concentrate on the pathologically narcissistic influences of parents on their children.

Thus Chapter III takes a detailed look at the narcissism of fathers. This chapter begins with an examination of the psychology of masculinity, which again provides a number of varying theories that tend to emphasize a shift from a primary concern with anatomy and biology to a focus on social and interpersonal influences. This section is followed by an attempt to develop an integrative model of masculinity and to take note of the expanding male identity as well as its conflicts and uncertainties. Then attention is devoted to the fathering process with an emphasis on the father's narcissism and how this can be used in both adaptive and maladaptive ways.

The narcissism of mothers is explored in Chapter IV, beginning with femininity which has been significantly reformulated in psychoanalytic theory. Developmental theories are reconsidered, including structural theory, differentiation, and connection, as well as integrated theories of female development. Emphasis is given to the complexity of the process and the role of narcissism which significantly contributes to contemporary views of gender identity for women as it also has for men. Roles are expanded, less definitive, and have greater potentials. Then the focus is placed on the mothering process which has such a powerful cultural connection with being a woman. Particular note is taken of the mother's narcissism in its facilitation or restriction of the psychological growth of children.

It is apparent in these chapters on fathers and mothers that development is an interactive process involving the entire family, and that influences occur between all members. Of particular interest is the process of negative interactions resulting in pathological narcissism. Thus the next chapter of the book looks at the development of specific disturbances within the context of pathological narcissism as a general construct for all psychological disorders. Up to this point the theories of pathological narcissism described have focused on what is often termed a "narcissistic disorder." In Chapter V the psychodynamics of pathological narcissism are given detailed consideration with particular attention paid to pathology that appears to be the result of caretaker-child interactions. These provide suggestions for psychodynamic patterns, but stress the subjectivity of pathology and the necessity for individualized genetic reconstructions. Narcissism as a personal perspective that can be used to understand a variety of psychopathologies is illustrated in psychosis, neurosis, and character disorders, specifically schizophrenia, depression, and borderline disorder. Clinical material is used to understand the role of narcissism in symptom manifestations, psychodynamics, and treatment procedures.

Chapter VI takes notice of the workings of narcissism as a personal perspective in the analytic hour and the supervisory hour. The emphasis is on the presence and the use of narcissism in therapists and in supervisors, with four segments each of therapy and supervisory sessions. In Chapter VII narcissism is explored in the context of tracing the evolution of psychoanalytic practice and theory in regard to the development of relationships. Two main themes are developed, namely a link between structural theory and separation, and a link between relational theory and connection. Both models are seen as expanding narcissism in significant ways, yet also limiting its potential. Separation reduces interpersonal influences, but limits subjectivity through instinctual and social-relational pressures. Connection decreases drive influences but emphasizes the relational context of subjectivity. It is suggested that a more effective approach is to build on the knowledge provided by the study of separation and connection to now emphasize the distinctiveness of subjects and the motivational power of narcissism rather than what influences it. This theme is amplified in the final chapter (VIII) where it is proposed that narcissism can be very effectively used as an organizing principle for the understanding of motivation, development, and psychoanalytic interventions. Thus a journey is completed from the origins of narcissism through its many meanings and usages to a contemporary view that stresses the power of subjectivity embodied in the concept of narcissism. The journey also includes a look at the continuing evolution of psychoanalysis from its structural roots to its current relational and interpersonal concerns that indeed highlights the diversity and creativity of psychoanalytic thought. It seems accurate to say that a reconstruction is under way, but at the moment what is unsettled is more striking than what can be definitively affirmed.

A number of people have been helpful in developing this book. First, I want to acknowledge Sheila Rouslin Welt who has been my co-author for previous books about narcissism. Then there are people who have had strong influences on my thinking, namely Rafael Javier, Frank Patalano, Lewis Aron, Stanley Teitelbaum, Clemens Loew, Sylvia Teitelbaum, Rose Oosting, the faculty at the Contemporary Center for Advanced Psychoanalytic Studies, and the members of my "for eternity" peer supervision group. I am indebted to Sonja Ramirez, Abigail Herron, Paul Bulman, and Bhupin Butaney for their technical support, and to St. John's University for the provision of time and resources to complete this book. Finally, I am especially grateful to Mary Jane Herron for the many stimulating discussions in which her "views from the Stone Center" were provocative additions to my knowledge base.

I
The Meaning of Narcissism

Narcissism seems to have achieved the unfortunate status of a hydra with so many meanings and developments that precision is limited and conceptual confusion abounds. The problematic status of narcissism has been noted in a series of reviews that have also stressed the possible values of the concept (Fiscalini, 1993; Moore, 1975; Pulver, 1970). It is my intention to try to realize this elusive potential of narcissism through an exploration of its motivational properties. In doing so I will first trace the development of narcissism from its origins as a psychoanalytic concept through its journey of definition and usages. In turn, this will provide the material to formulate a working description of narcissism as a core motivational force.

The Birth of Narcissism

Freud (1914) is usually credited with the significant introduction of narcissism to the language of psychoanalysis, although he had acknowledged precursors such as Nacke, Havelock Ellis, and Sadger. The concept of narcissism was derived from the myth of Narcissus, which has more than one version and numerous interpretations. As a result the myth may be seen as primarily portending the future of the concept, but having more limited value as a guide to the precise meaning of narcissism. Narcissus was distinguished by his beauty, but he would only continue living if he did not look upon his own features for an extended period of time. Either he fell in love with his own reflection in the water (the most frequent version) or he was fixedly recalling the features of a beloved twin sister that would appear to be projected into his own image in the water (or at least was imagined in proximity to his image). Narcissus had a history of spurning the love of others, including the nymph Echo, who could only repeat whatever Narcissus said to himself. In all versions he died because he apparently did little but look at and listen to himself. If love for another was present, it was merged into love for an image of himself.

The behavior of Narcissus has been interpreted as extreme example of objectlessness and self-admiration, as well as an example of pathological object relations and death by self-neglect (Auerbach, 1993). It is clear that a certain type of inner involvement, as opposed to relating to the external world, was a fatal way to live. Thus narcissism, via the myth, could be construed as deadly pathological behavior, and it was as a perversion that its originators described it. After death, Narcissus was transformed into a beautiful flower, the white narcissus, which had the power to relieve pain. If the emphasis is on pathology, then the numbing aspect is emphasized, but the assuaging aspect is also there, along with the beauty of the flower for whomever gazes upon it. As a result, the symbolism of the flower raises the possibility of a mixed outcome, positive and negative features, which were incorporated into Freud's subsequent conception of narcissism.

Although Freud's predecessors considered narcissism to be a perversion, and he also saw its applicability in that context, for Freud narcissism was something much more encompassing. Such a view is congruent with the many interpretations of the myth (Bach, 1985; Bergmann, 1987; Rosenman, 1981; Spotnitz & Resnikoff, 1954), but Freud was not that literal about myths, instead using them as starting points for broader ideas which he then viewed as grounded in clinical/theoretical evidence rather than in the myths.

Given that the evidence gathering went on over time, and that for Freud the evidence was often more inferential than directly observational, it is quite understandable that narcissism always had certain shifting conceptual aspects. Essentially, Freud viewed narcissism as self-involvement that was likely to have both normal and pathological manifestations in all people. He did contrast it rather sharply with regard for others, to the point that object love posed a threat to self esteem. Narcissism was divided into primary, an undifferentiated objectless state, and secondary, where after having had to invest energy in objects outside the self due to frustration with attempts to maintain autoerotic gratification, it was necessary to restore the self by recapturing the energy from the objects. Because psychic preservation of the self required energy that was of limited quantity, object cathexis was a secondary preference to self-cathexis. Thus, the self would either have to withdraw love from objects or get object love without giving it, or give it in such a way that it was experienced as self love whenever the self needed additional psychic energy to maintain self-esteem. At the same time, object relations were considered necessary and desired for need satisfaction, as well as being expedient due to the dependent nature of all individuals. Given the economic concept of a fixed quantity of psychic energy per individual, a balancing act appeared perpetually necessary, and others' needs would appear to be at a loss in relation to narcissistic needs. Although narcissism contained healthy self-love, such narcissism could move into opposition to loving another. In fact, this was a likely situation, even with the existence of civilizing defenses such as sublimation, as well as structures such as the super-ego which could have a socializing effect on the instincts as well as offering the ego ideal for self-esteem.

In Freud's initial formulations (1911, 1913, 1914), autoerotism preceded narcissism as the beginning developmental stage. Autoerotism is the first phase of libidinal organization in which the infant's body is cathected, whereas object love follows narcissism. Narcissism comes about through the development of the ego, which adds the ability to form an image of one's body. Narcissism at this point was depicted as a libidinal cathexis of the ego, although the ego at the time was often used interchangeably with the self, and here refers to a body ego. Also, such a conception involved excessively valuing the self and in turn the creation of an ego ideal.

Auerbach (1993) notes that Freud fluctuated to some degree from the idea of development beginning with an objectless state, and at times saw autoerotism as coming after a self-preservative object cathexis. However, in establishing the structural model (Freud, 1923), primary narcissism became the first stage of development, and autoerotism became part of narcissism. Primary narcissism was characterized by a lack of differentiation so that there was both a lack of awareness of objects and a corresponding lack of investment of energy in them. However, there is also some confusion here because the infant was viewed as using hallucinatory wish-fulfillment to gratify needs, which in turn posits an object image based on some type of object awareness. The discovery of objects was depicted as depending on frustration, namely the inability to maintain apparently autoerotic gratification, and engenders initial hostility toward objects because of the personal libidinal depletion involved in object cathexis.

The way Freud's economic model was structured makes it difficult to integrate self-love and love for others. The latter looks especially tenuous, fragile, and paradoxically selfish, lacking the mutuality and permanence that many people experience. If narcissism was to be equated with self-love, then there would have to be a type of narcissism that permitted self-love and object-love to coexist in a reasonable, clinically based, realistic way. There is room for that with self-regard or self-esteem being components of narcissism, but the type of coexistence just described is difficult to discern because Freud's emphasis was on the quantity of psychic energy involved. Thus, as Fiscalini (1993) notes, the sorting out of quality in Freud's model is complex. Auerbach (1993) indicates that quantity was applied to the lack of investment in objects as a defining characteristic of narcissism, whereas quality was reflected in the idea of unawareness of objects. The quantity issue, including the very existence of psychic energy, was the source of much initial debate, while the quality got considerable agreement as a concept of undifferentiation, although that too would change. There is a need to soften the oppositional flavor of narcissism by bringing the concept into line with the observable realities of self-love and object-love, and this need was left unfilled in Freud's theorizing.

However, Freud's work on narcissism had a considerable, enduring impact on the entire psychoanalytic field. As Sandler, Person, and Fonagy (1991) note in their retrospective view, Freud's essay on narcissism was the start of a lengthy discussion. In that introduction the foundation was provided for structural theory, ego psychology, relational theory and self psychology, through consideration of the ego, ego ideal, conscience, self, self-regard, internalization, identification, object choice, sublimation, and relational motivations. The normality of narcissism was presented, along with its pathology in schizophrenia, perversion, homosexuality, organic disease, and hypochondria. In particular, the faults of excessive narcissism were highlighted, including the narcissistic attitude as a resistance to treatment. Freud's legacy for narcissism itself was the presence of an important, vital, complex, and confusing construct that needed work.

Ego Psychology

The development and role of the ego became focal in psychoanalysis. Part of this ego-emphasis was a redefinition of narcissism "as the libidinal cathexis not of the ego but of the self" (Hartmann, 1950, p.127). This clarified the structure of the ego by making narcissism an investment in the self-representation within the ego. This cathexis was generally thought of as libidinal, although the possibility existed of a parallel aggressive cathexis (Moore, 1975).

The ego was also viewed as having an adaptive function and being inborn, a product of an undifferentiated matrix from which structures differentiate and capacities develop. The economic principle was expanded to permit energy conversion for adaptive purposes, thus lessening the oppositional duality of narcissism and object love. The developmental process involved gradual formations of self and object representations in the service of adaptation, which in turn was the maintenance of an equilibrium between the organism and its environment.

However, the shift of cathexis from the ego to the self-representation within the ego still left confusion about the origination of narcissism. Hartmann (1950) noted the value in distinguishing between ego, self, and personality in order to develop a clear concept of narcissism, but a major difficulty lies in defining the self, which at this point was described as the person distinct from the object. That person is known by its internal representation, but that person also exists from conception in some form, so where and when does narcissism originate?

Speigel (1959) took note of the complications surrounding the term "self," in particular using self to designate the total person (and the total mind) as well as using it to denote self representations as distinct from object representations in one mind. He suggests using self to refer to all representations of the self as distinct from the object representations, whereas person is the broad concept of the total physical and mental being. Self is then a subdivision of the person, a representational image of the "I."

The need for that image then calls into question the existence of narcissism in states of undifferentiation (Jacobson, 1954). Nonetheless, the idea of an objectless or preobjectal state that existed from birth until the discovery of the self and the object world was generally equated with primary narcissism (Jacobson, 1964; Mahler, 1968; Spitz, 1965). One explanation for this is that the term is being used descriptively, as in the observation of autoerotic activity, as contrasted with metapsychologically to refer to energy distribution. Another possibility is that there was a shift from the emphasis on the economics of drive discharge to a metapsychology of attitude and affects (Joffe & Sandler, 1968). Such a shift involves increasing the importance of affects and object relations at the same time that it maintains a concern with drive discharge (Kernberg, 1984).

Interest in narcissistic pathology places an emphasis on narcissism as a constellation of pathological characteristics that are in varying degrees opposed to object love. Narcissism then appears as a deficit state, or a series of defensive operations, shifting the focus away from the economic principle, although this view assumes some type of self structure which has the deficit and/or the defense. In essence, either the economic principle is slighted, ignored, or treated selectively so that primary narcissism becomes the objectless or preobjectal state of the early months of life and secondary narcissism appears with self and object differentiation. The primary-secondary distinction appears less frequently and narcissism is depicted primarily as self-interest in comparison with object interest, including a quantitative difference between narcissistic libido and object libido.

The shifts in how narcissism was described and used are noted by Moore (1975). The many meanings of narcissism included a developmental stage, a type of libido or object choice, an attitude or affect, systems and processes, and a personality type. After reviewing the literature on narcissism up to 1975, Moore concludes that it is best to accept its complexity and define it in context when it is employed, assuming that the meaning can be conveyed accurately in specific instances.

Pulver (1970) has a different view, having also reviewed similar literature on narcissism. First he notes that a distinction needs to be made between narcissism as a metapsychological concept and as a term for specific psychic phenomena. By the time Freud's 1914 paper on narcissism was completed, narcissism had been used to describe a sexual perversion (one's body as a sexual object), a developmental stage (libidinal cathexis of the ego), types of object relationships (object choice based on self-identification, lack of object relations), and components of self-regard (self-esteem). One reaction was to suggest restricting the term to aspects of self-esteem (Joffe & Sandler, 1967). Healthy narcissism is high self-esteem from pleasurable affect-self-representation connections, whereas pathological narcissism is defensive self-idealization. However, selecting any one of the major descriptions of narcissism and eliminating or renaming the others was generally seen as too restrictive, and Pulver (1970) offered a compromise. He suggested renaming a type of narcissism that was applied to minimal self-interest, but retained the idea of narcissism as a relatively broad concept referring to some aspects of the self. At the same time, greater specificity was suggested whenever possible.

The revisions by Pulver (1970) and Moore (1975) primarily make it clear that narcissism was undergoing widespread application, but clarity was decreasing for a concept that from the start had been confusing. Furthermore, the attempts to develop more precision are not that satisfactory, emphasizing the complexity of narcissism. In addition to these developments there were shifts away from economic perspectives and from the primacy of drives, towards affects and objects, as well as greater usage and description of the structure "self."

For example, the libidinal target of narcissism became the self (Hartmann, 1950), which in turn was viewed as a representation of the total person (self-representation) within the ego (Jacobson, 1964). Attention was given to the differentiation of self- and object representations, and the role of identification, internalization, and ego functions involved in structuralization, as well as the differentiation and structuralization of the drives. The distinction was drawn between internalized object relations and external object relations, and it was suggested that libido invested in self and objects was more likely to be enhancing to both than mutually exclusive (Kernberg, 1975; Schafer, 1968). More radical changes were seen in the distinction made between the self as structure and the self as experience (Kohut, 1971a; Modell, 1968), and alternatives to Hartmann's definition of narcissism (Kohut, 1971b; Murray, 1964; Stolorow, 1975). However, these departures from mainstream theoretical alterations remained connected to a conceptual ego psychological framework, and Hartmann's definition of narcissism tended to prevail.

At the same time, as Teicholz (1978) pointed out, this definition was problematic and required different meanings for the terms used in the definition, particularly libido and self, as well as reformulations of the roles of related concepts, such as the ego, ego ideal, and self-esteem. For example, if the drives are viewed as a modifiable duality of libido and aggression, then narcissism involves relatively fused libidinal and aggressive drives (libido dominates) that are neutralized and integrated, rather than solely libido. The ego-ideal, generally viewed as a component of the superego, appears as the standard of the ideal self for the self-representation, and begins with feelings of omnipotence prior to self and object differentiation that are subject to differentiation and structuralization that include object relations and identifications. Of particular interest are the degrees of self-idealization and object idealization in forming the self-representation. Through a comparative evaluation between the self-representation and the ego-ideal a cognitive-affective attitude toward the self is developed representing self-esteem. On that basis then, narcissism was often equated with the positive or negative evaluation of the self that in turn comprised self-esteem, and disturbances to the latter affected the former. Thus pathological narcissism can result from unstable or unrealistic self-representations, or ego defects, or superego deficiencies, or the lack of drive fusion or drive neutralization. These disturbances result in affects, such as anxiety or depression, that result in defenses, symptoms, and/or character pathology that is described as narcissistic (Teicholz, 1978).

Etchegoyen (1991) has pointed out that self-esteem has three sources, infantile narcissism, the ego-ideal, and satisfaction of object-libido, so it is also necessary in understanding the meaning of narcissism to look more closely at the role of object relations. The focus on self-esteem, however, does make the point that although narcissism at this time was still being described as a libidinal investment of the self, this was often translated as meaning an attitude about the self. This meaning was actually broadened into an attitude about the self and others. Thus current ego psychological theory describes the relationship between self representations and object representations in terms of a narcissistic balance or imbalance, depending on whether both are evenly valued, or one is overvalued at the expense of the other (Blanck & Blanck, 1994).

In determining the nature of narcissism as it is expressed in relation to objects it is necessary to consider more than observable object relations because each person has an internalized set of object representations and representations of the relations between self and the internalized objects. These are self representations in the sense that the self is their agent, but they are about others, or others and the self, yet they reflect narcissism. In addition, representations are primarily derived from types of identifications, as well as through separation of the self from others. Thus narcissism appears in a relational context that at the same time emphasizes the role of the self in object relations.

Teicholz (1978) summarizes the consensus of opinion about narcissism at that time by stressing ego development in terms of differentiated and integrated self- and object representations, optimally gratifying parenting, and drive development, including neutralization and transformation. Difficulties in any of these areas is pictured as promoting pathological narcissism in terms of omnipotent self and object images or a distorted ego-ideal. She concludes by calling for the development of a broader definition of narcissism, especially including the role of the drives, self- and object representations, the ego-ideal, and the ego functions of perception, judgement, synthesis, and neutralization. Unfortunately, there is a sense in such a conclusion that the unique value of narcissism is starting to get lost, that normal narcissism is being equated with normal self functioning, and in turn may be an unnecessary term. This is undoubtedly not what was intended, but it suggests a background for viewing the term "narcissistic" as most distinct and useful when describing a type of pathology. However, before viewing pathological narcissism, it is useful to look at the dissenters whose work ultimately became very influential in understanding the value of narcissism.

Stolorow and Kohut
        Stolorow suggested the following description of narcissism: "Mental activity is narcissistic to the degree that its function is to maintain the structural cohesiveness, temporal stability, and positive affective colouring of the self-representations" (1975, p.179).
        His reasons for this type of definition are the limitations of the economic model and drive theory and the vagueness of the terms self and libido. He considers it a functional definition in keeping with ego psychology's emphasis on multiple functions served by specific mental activities. Support for the definition is derived from the distinction made by Hartmann (1950) between ego, self, and self-representations, as well as Jacobson (1964) describing narcissism as the libidinal cathexis of the self-representation, and even Freud (1914) implying that the function of narcissistic object choice is the regulation of self-esteem. Reich (1953,1960) is credited with being the first to clearly show how narcissistic patterns maintain the self-representation. Kohut (1971a) is given particular attention because of his emphasis on internal structures that maintain self-cohesiveness and self-esteem, although Kohut is seen at this time as still maintaining the connection between narcissism and an economic model.
        Stolorow (1975) also indicates that there does not have to be an antithesis between narcissism and object relationships because object relationships can serve narcissistic functions, namely maintenance of stability, cohesiveness, and positive affect of the self-representation. Also, he views the earliest neonatal stage as undifferentiated symbiotic

fusion (neither primary narcissism nor primary object relatedness) preceding self-object differentiation. The earliest object relationships serve the narcissistic function of consolidating a basic self-representation with limited existing stability and cohesiveness. There is a developmental line of narcissism from primitive prestructural object relations towards higher forms of narcissism through gradual growth of internal structures whose functions maintain self-representations. Narcissism is differentiated from self-esteem, which is described as a complex, multiply determined affective state which narcissism services when necessary to restore, repair, stabilize, or protect self-esteem. The healthy or unhealthy aspects of narcissism are determined by the degree to which self-representation maintenance is successful. Stolorow also suggests that an understanding of the function of narcissism can increase empathy and reduce countertransference in the therapeutic process because it clarifies the necessity of narcissistic operations for patients.

Stolorow's description of narcissism retains some of the problems of the definition it seeks to supplant. For example, structural cohesiveness and temporal stability of the self-representations are not specifically defined. In the beginning of the paper the positive affective colouring of the self-representations appears to be equated with self-esteem, but later in the paper, that aspect of the self-representation appears to be only part of self-esteem. Also, although he frequently cites Kohut's work in support of the functional definition of narcissism, he does not redefine the self to bring that concept in accord with Kohut's view, but instead retains Hartmann's conception of the self, which is strongly tied to the economic model Stolorow wishes to replace.

These omissions are of significance because in Stolorow's subsequent work he clearly favors Kohut's views about the self, so it is probable that such a shift is implied. It is also possible to hypothesize that his views of self cohesion and stability are primarily in accord with Kohut's, although Stolorow has derided the reification of constructs such as "the self" and emphasized intersubjectivity as the most accurate way to understand behavior (Stolorow & Atwood, 1992).

Eagle (1984) provides critical comments in regard to both Stolorow's concept of healthy narcissism and the lack of reciprocity between narcissism and object libido. Eagle argues that defining narcissism as healthy or pathological in terms of successful self-maintenance and self-enhancement causes narcissistic exploitation to be viewed as healthy as long as it works, and realistic drops in self-esteem to be erroneously viewed as pathological. However, it could be argued that the characteristics of narcissistic disorders are illusions of self-enhancement, and that realistic drops in self-esteem are illusions of self-disparagement, and not at all what Stolorow had in mind.

Beyond that, though, Eagle asserts that self-maintenance is often a by-product of goals, values, ambitions, and object-directed interests, rather than self-maintenance motivating them. Thus, considerable room is made for autonomous pursuits that are independent of narcissism because they are not seen as motivated by self-enhancement. However, the motives that Eagle assigns for these behaviors are "the interest they arouse and the enjoyment and gratification they provide" (1984, p.57). Such motives have a self-referent, namely they create something positive for the self in that their satisfaction is a self-satisfaction, and thus self-maintaining or self-enhancing. As a result the assertions and evidence presented in their support do not appear as a convincing refutation of healthy narcissism.

Eagle also contends that a lack of an adversarial relationship between narcissism and object relatedness is more apparent than real because of the quality of object relations. A distinction is thereby drawn between narcissistic object relations and object-directed relationships which seems to be a continuation of the theme of the necessary lack of healthy narcissism. No room is allowed for the possibility that all relationships are interactive, or as Stolorow would ultimately suggest, intersubjective, and in that sense a mixture of narcissistic and object libido.

Eagle concludes that healthy narcissism, if the term is to be used, refers to limited narcissism, but now he seems to have returned to missing the quality of narcissism and emphasizing the quantity. In fact, without stating it in Freud's economy of psychic energy terms, he agrees with Freud in believing that self-absorption limits genuine concern for others. Thus self-direction is contrasted with object-direction, yet again this view makes self-direction unidimensional as opposed to the possibility that one could be motivated to enhance the self by being genuinely interested in others. Narcissism is being restricted by Eagle and expanded by Stolorow, with Freud providing the groundwork for each of them with both the reciprocity principle and the idea of normal narcissism.

What is particularly striking about Storolow's change in the definition of narcissism is the direction he was moving, namely, the abandonment of the economic view and of libido as it was customarily known, in order to develop a significantly more relational perspective. Although framed at that time in terms of ego psychology, the functional emphasis of Storolow, particularly in regard to using an understanding of the function of narcissism as a way for the therapist to reduce countertransference and increase empathy, illustrates how the consideration of narcissism sparks the development of other significant concepts.

Freud, for example, used his works on narcissism as a way to open up consideration of the ego and the development of structural theory. This in turn was followed by the development of ego psychology and attempts to view narcissism in ego psychological terms. Stolorow began as ostensibly part of the ego psychological emphasis, although his subsequent formulations of an intersubjective emphasis is more in accord with the interpersonal and object relations movements that were paralleling ego psychology.

Kohut (1971a) initially proposed a psychology of the self that was apparently designed to compliment existing psychoanalytic theory, and contained a separate line of development for narcissism which begins with autoerotism and a fragmented self and culminates in a cohesive self. Within the developmental process an exhibitionistic and grandiose self is established through empathetic mirroring and parental idealization. These early forms of grandiosity and idealization are modified and transformed into healthy narcissism that includes a cohesive self with adequate self-esteem and ambition, ideals and values. Structural development takes place through the withdrawal of narcissistic cathexis from selfobjects and subsequent internalization so that the child takes over selfobject functions. This process is described as transmuting internalizations that involve shifts in relating to the self and others. Relationships begin with others as selfobjects who are relied on to carry out essential functions, such as self-cohesiveness, and moves into experiencing others as separate as well as into independent actions. Narcissistic pathology results primarily from parental failures in providing mirroring and idealization opportunities.

Initially, Kohut viewed the self as part of the ego, and he used words such as libido and cathexis that appeared to maintain a bridge to the then prevalent ego psychology. Self psychology was first proposed as applicable to preoedipal stages and the development and pathology of narcissism, with the drive theory applicable to oedipal stages and neurotic conflicts. However, Kohut (1977, 1984) subsequently expanded the scope of self psychology so that it became a general psychoanalytic theory of development in which drives and impulse gratification are considered secondary to the self and relational development with the self as a superordinate structure. Psychosexual stages and object relations stages are essentially replaced by stages in the development of the self. These stages were originally framed in terms of the development of narcissism, but later on this was downplayed in favor of self-maintenance, self-cohesion, and self-enhancement.

Ornstein (1991) points out that Kohut viewed narcissism as the normal nutrient for building structure, so that pathology becomes a matter of disturbances in the self structure (deficits, defenses) that come from inadequate narcissistic investments. Inevitable failures to provide support for the maintenance of narcissism result in the development of the grandiose self and the omnipotent idealized object which will be converted into both self-esteem (a narcissistic component of the superego) and mature selfobject relations. Primacy is given to deficits in meeting mirroring and idealizing needs, with conflicts arising secondarily due to these deficits.

Ornstein (1991) notes that narcissism was left behind as self psychology expanded to the bipolar self (self-assertive and idealizing) which was the dominant structure. Eagle (1984) however sees narcissism as embedded in Kohut's work, and takes issue with a number of his propositions, such as an inevitable early phase of grandiosity, and particularly, his concept of healthy narcissism. Kohut is particularly clear and forceful about the latter, stating, "I have, of course, taken an in essence affirmative attitude toward narcissism" (1971b, p.363).

Eagle (1984) cites three meanings of narcissism as reflected in its current usage, namely the lack of differentiation between self and others, the regulation of self-esteem, and self-absorption. Self-absorption may be congruent with Kohut's contention that object-directed pursuits are in service of the self, but Eagle considers narcissism and object interest to be singularly distinct, thereby moving narcissism primarily into the category of pathology. In this attempt to clear away the conceptual fog that exists when narcissism is viewed broadly, replacement terms would have to be used to describe healthy narcissism, such as a sense of adequacy or self-esteem. Thus the question is repeatedly raised as to whether it is possible to effectively retain Freud's original conception of narcissism as a term that embraced health and pathology.

Also, Bacal and Newman (1990) assert that self psychology has a relational core, and that raises the possibility of relations as essentially self-enhancing or narcissistic without implying pathology. In turn that moves the concept in the other direction, meaning other terms for narcissistic pathology, such as vanity, conceit, and alienation. In addition, the trend toward the intersubjective emphasizes experience, and by doing so blurs a distinction between concepts such as self-interest and object-interest. Instead the idea of selfobject relations at all developmental levels is emphasized.

Relational Theorists
Although Bacal and Newman (1990) offer a self psychology context for relational theories, self psychology has been far more definitive about its embrace of narcissism than most relational theories. In the main, relational theorists talked about the concept by using words other than narcissism, and were prone to view the word as synonymous with some form of relational disturbance. For example, Suttie (1935) disputed the existence of primary narcissism, instead describing an initial undifferentiated phase as infantile solipsism that is followed by object cathexis. He invested the infant with a capacity for relatedness that contrasted with narcissism, which he viewed as a turning into the self due to disrupted object relationships. Balint (1968) began the developmental cycle with primary object love which is inevitably disrupted. One possible reaction to the disruption is that the child uses narcissism to try to give the self what had been experienced in relation to the object, in turn making narcissism a defensive reaction to the lack or limit of an object relation.

Narcissism as pathological is made explicit by Bacal and Newman (1991) when they depict narcissism as describing either a disorder or an apparently self-syntonic state which is actually unstable. In order to establish congruence with a self-psychological context for relational theories, they translate Kohut's narcissism into the need for phase appropriate selfobject functioning, and reserve the term "narcissistic" for disturbances in normal self-selfobject relationships that result in injuries to the self. This shifts the view of pathological narcissism as self-centeredness defending against object love to an arrest in the development of the self, but it avoids the issue of healthy narcissism, which apparently would be called something other than narcissism.

Fiscalini (1993) makes the point that cultural-interpersonal theorists have had considerable interest in narcissism, and that some did make use of the term. Two examples are Horney and Fromm, both of whom viewed narcissism as self-alienation. Horney (1950) considered narcissism to be self-inflation, and Fromm (1964) described a narcissistic orientation that ranged from moderate self-centeredness to grandiosity. Then using different language, Sullivan (1940) described a number of personality types that could be considered narcissistic, namely self-absorbed, ambition-ridden, inadequate, and chronically adolescent. Frequently interpersonal theorists have discussed narcissism in terms of self-regard, self-idealization, grandiosity, idealization, and detachment.

Fiscalini (1993) also noted that recently, in an attempt to bridge the language gap with other schools of psychoanalytic thought, relational theorists have devoted explicit attention to narcissism. The purpose is to integrate material about problems of self-development, and the emphasis is on narcissism as a form of pathology of the self. The types of self experience or the dimensions of the self that have been included under the rubric of narcissism are self-esteem, self-absorption (self-extension and self-centeredness), self-inflation, and self-perfection.

Within the framework of pathological narcissism there is disagreement as to the range of disturbances that are covered by narcissism. Horney (1950) appears predictive in her broad description of neuroses that emphasized defensive self-idealization, self-alienation, and compensatory grandiosity because Kohut ultimately depicts all disorders as pathology of the self. In contrast, Kernberg (1975) describes a specific narcissistic personality disorder. The latter view has prevailed in official diagnostic classifications, although with continuing debate as to specific characteristics that predates Kohut's 1968 introduction of the term "narcissistic personality disorder" (Rothstein, 1979).

Kernberg's narcissists and Kohut's narcissists share grandiosity, but Kernberg sees the grandiosity as defensive with a coexisting sense of inferiority derived from cold, unempathetic parenting. The deprivation is reinforced by projected rages. A grandiose self is defensively developed from a merger of admired aspects of the child and fantasies of the self and loving parents. Treatment stresses interpretation of the defensive grandiosity and repairing split self-representations, with aggression as a major etiological stimulus. The formulation is aimed at specific pathology, primarily grandiosity, emptiness, exploration of others, chronic envy, and a lack of values. In contrast, Kohut views the narcissistic disorder as arrested development, with narcissistic rage as primarily reactive, and with narcissistic disturbances broadly applicable as manipulations of problematic self-object relations.

The majority approach seems to favor the view of a specific narcissistic personality disorder, although Kohut's conceptions continue to be apparent, particularly the emphasis on the self. For example, Bach (1985) describes the self experientially as people's theories about themselves, and in this context views the narcissistic disorder as deficits in self-perception, organization of language and thought, volition, mood, and the perception of space, time, and causality. Akhtar and Anderson (1982) reviewed descriptions of the narcissistic personality and suggested clinical features that concerned self-concept, interpersonal relations, social adaptation, ideals, sexuality, and cognitive style. DSM IV (American Psychiatric Association, 1994) emphasizes a pattern of grandiosity, need for admiration, and a lack of empathy.

Fiscalini (1993) suggests a constellation of grandiosity, self-centeredness, contempt and idealization of the self and others, vulnerable self-esteem, psychological inaccessibility, entitlement, need for admiration, and coerciveness. He suggests that all people are narcissistic in that they have problems with self-esteem and develop narcissistic defenses such as self-centeredness and grandiosity to varying degrees. Narcissism is seen as varying in severity, patterning, chronicity, and breadth, with narcissistic problems developing from interpersonal interactions, namely faulty parent-child relatedness. Specific etiological patterns are the shamed child, the spoiled child, and the special child, with the self-respecting child exemplifying healthy narcissism. The latter is the result of caretaking that provides for gradual reductions in the child's egocentricity, grandiosity, and idealization. Although this view allows for healthy narcissism, it prefers the use of narcissism as a description of problems in self-development. The self is also an interpersonal one, different from Kohut's self and self-objects, so that primacy is given to the relational environment, in essence moving away from narcissism based on a process of balancing reflections from others about the self. This appears to highlight a distinction between relational theories of the development of the self and self psychology. Although self psychology is relational in that the development of the self requires self-objects, relations are in service of the self much as they are in service of drives in drive theory. As a result narcissism is more of an obstacle in relational theory where the self is primarily object directed, and in turn, narcissism is experienced as more appropriate to pathology than growth of the self. If the infant is considered relational at birth, which is being suggested more frequently (Stern, 1985), and states such as normal autism and normal symbiosis, which were once equated with primary narcissism, are ruled out, the tendency may be to consider the degree to which the infant is not relational as narcissistic. This puts narcissism primarily in the pathological category because it opposes object relations to self-relations.

Shifting narcissism to a descriptive and/or explanatory term for pathology as contrasted to the broader usage is, as even its proponents admit, not that likely to gain widespread acceptance (Fiscalini, 1993). Historical usage works against it, as does the complexity of narcissism that makes substitutes for any of its significant aspects seem incomplete. Also, despite understandable dissatisfaction with the original economic theory of narcissism, any reformulation that narrows the concept, particularly when self and object relations are seen as being in opposition, could be construed as an economic theory. As a result, it appears useful to continue the search for reformulations of narcissism that may result in clarity yet preserve the unique complexity.

Reformulations

Although self psychology has been the most focused on healthy narcissism, another example is found in restricting narcissism to variations in self-esteem, viewed as an interactive concept involving drive satisfactions, object relations, and adaptation (Dare & Holder, 1981). This shift in emphasis is useful in promoting an understanding of the self-regard aspect of narcissism, but the integration of the mixture of concepts that has been assigned to narcissism remains difficult. This problem also appears when narcissism is described in terms of interactive dimensions that have been empirically validated, as vulnerability-sensitivity and grandiosity-exhibitionism (Wink, 1991) or the four dimensions of egocentrism, self-esteem, self-representation, and investment in others (Weston, 1990). The components that are being delineated actually emphasize the complexity of narcissism.

Bach (1985) approaches narcissism as a particular state of consciousness which can be a deficit and/or a defense. The state of consciousness is considered an organizing principle for self-awareness which has a range from sensory-motor non-awareness through differentiation of self and other to reflective self-awareness which evaluates and integrates the relationship of self to other. Reflective self-awareness is established through object relations that provide the experience of how others see the world and see the self, so that the relativity of the self is experienced and understood. The normal person establishes an equilibrium where the self and object world can be experienced as real, and relatively stable yet intermingled, with an ease of transition from one to the other. However, the narcissistic person has a different kind of experience in which there is either an overcathexis of the self or of the object world. In the former there is elation and grandiosity as well as fears of object loss and the loss of reality so that the subject and object become one. In the latter, there is depression, depersonalization and the self has been absorbed by the other. This representational framework also takes into account the role of drives in development, as well as emphasizing the perspective of ego psychology in objective self-awareness (self as an object among other objects as well as self among other selves) and the perspective of self psychology in subjective self-awareness (the self as the center of feeling, thought, and action), with the etiology of narcissistic disorders being primarily relational. Johnson (1987) also favors a relational etiology, but has a Reichian emphasis that makes narcissism primarily a disturbance of the body self, as well as stressing subjective awareness rather than the integration of subjective and objective self-awareness. As with Bach (1985), narcissism is considered primarily a form of pathology with disturbances of the self, language, thought, intentionality, time sense, and mood.

Auerbach (1993) builds on the work of Bach in regard to the role of narcissism in self-awareness. He uses findings from recent infant research that support the early development of a presymbolic representational capacity and the construction of a core self between two and six months. The core self includes agency, coherence, affectivity, and memory in rudimentary forms. Infants appear to enter the world with some awareness and interest in their environment, including their caretakers. Although differentiation between self and others increases with maturation, there is a lack of evidence for initial objectlessness, normal autism, fusion, normal symbiosis, and fantasies of omnipotence. Some of these concepts become untenable because of the degree of infant awareness that does appear to exist starting at birth, if not before, as well as corresponding attachment to objects, whereas others become unreasonable, such as fantasies, because they require symbolic thought and language that is not in place in infancy. Auerbach (1993) contends that infants have sufficient awareness and interest in others to refute the idea of an extreme self-focus in the early weeks/months of life, but they lack sufficient cognitive and affective ability to form fantasies of infantile omnipotence. Although there is not a phase without objects, the pace of differentiation is such that the self-representation is not considered to be in place until the second year of life. Thus, narcissism cannot be considered to refer to an objectless state, which now appears to never exist, but narcissism appears only when there are capacities for self-recognition and for considering oneself as separate from others. Narcissistic disorders then are disturbances in the representations of self and others.

Self-representation involves an integration of subjective and objective perspectives about the self, a reflexive self-awareness that can result in conflict based on perceived differences between the real and ideal selves. Auerbach (1993) considers narcissism as the illusion of a unitary self to defend against self-reflexive conflicts. Shame is depicted as the core affect for narcissism, with prereflective shame proceeding objective self-awareness, and reflective shame producing narcissistic illusions. Both self-enhancement and self-effacement can be used to avoid objective self-awareness and create a sense of oneness for the self. Although narcissistic personality disorders can evoke cohesive self-images, they cannot make a smooth transition between subjective and objective forms of self-awareness (Bach, 1985).

Auerbach's approach is to view narcissism as primarily pathological, but operating in a range that includes normality, as for example from a biased self-enhancement to grandiosity. He suggests a number of limitations, such as not explaining narcissism in people with relative representational stability and insufficient explanation of reflexive self-awareness throughout the life cycle. In terms of explaining the meaning of narcissism, the problems are that it does restrict narcissism to pathology, and that it also restricts the pathological mechanism to a defensive illusion appearing only when there is a self-reflexive conflict.

Narcissism as an illusion, and basically a defense, has been suggested by others in different contexts. Rothstein (1984) suggests the illusion of a perfect self fused with a perfect object to avoid the loss of an original state of felt perfection in symbiosis. Kohut (1971a) considers illusions of grandeur and idealization as normal developmental features. Becker (1973) views narcissism as an illusion of complete self-sufficiency based on a need to deny mortality. Mitchell (1988) suggests a dialectic approach to narcissism in which healthy narcissism represents a balance between illusion and reality. New illusions are developed and dissolved as reality dictates, whereas in pathological narcissism illusions prevail. These illusions tend to be categorized into grandiosity, idealization, and fusion, which in turn appear to be the ingredients of narcissism. Bromberg (1983) considers narcissistic individuals to be developmentally fixed between reflected self-appraisal and a disguised search for such an appraisal, without a sense of full involvement in life. These people are caught up in a self-image of perfection that always has to be protected, and are particularly vulnerable to any recognition of dependency needs.

Auerbach (1993) notes that the vulnerability may be defended against by variations in self-esteem ranging from self-enhancement to self-effacement. In the former, shame is reduced through an illusory self-sufficiency, whereas in the latter subjectivity is obscured by an illusory merger, both reflecting difficulties in making transitions between subjective and objective self-awareness.

Bromberg (1983) indicates that the relational emphasis in psychoanalysis supports a view of narcissistic pathology that is described as attempts to preserve the structural stability of the self-representation, as well as protecting and maintaining the experience of the well-being of the self. The self is then being maintained by remaining developmentally fixated in terms of emotional and interpersonal growth. The fixation is viewed as primarily the result of faulty parenting, although Auerbach (1993) points out that the interaction between constitutional and environmental factors is unknown in regard to specific causality, and that empirical evidence is lacking for either preoedipal or oedipal conflicts necessarily producing narcissistic character pathology. Clinical observations are therefore the primary evidence, and these mainly support a genesis of parental errors or failures in the preoedipal period. The facilitation of growth is in turn believed to be facilitated if an environment is developed which aids the integration of accurate self-experience within an interpersonal self-representation.

Fine (1986) reviewed a number of these reformulations and noted their emphasis on one or more aspects of the original constellation that was designed as narcissism. There has been both an increase in connotations, as well as a restriction in meaning in order to develop a focus, with the net result of making it increasingly difficult to define narcissism. Fine prefers that narcissism be defined as self-involvement, without positive or negative connotations, and that the self be described in a common sense manner. However, such a definition of narcissism does not obviate some of the difficulties already noted, particularly the issue of whether the self is to be equated with the total person or with the self-representation, which as an image of the person is only a part of the total person. Also at issue is when the self comes into being because that is usually considered the point of entry for narcissism, and, based on the evidence reviewed, this could vary between birth and the second year of life. Then, the use of "self-involvement" suggests an opposition of the self to object involvement, although it is difficult to describe the state of the self in terms other than in relation to objects without falling prey to what Stolorow and Atwood term "the myth of the isolated mind" (1992, p.7).

Conclusions

The work of the authors cited in this chapter make it apparent that narcissism is particularly complex. Any definition that has been suggested can be subject to criticism, usually because something is neglected, but if any extremely comprehensive definition was offered, it could be met with the criticism that its breadth restricts its utility. Narrowing the definition has been the favored approach, and then it is talked about more often as a negative trait rather than a positive or neutral one. The authors emphasizing the equation between narcissism and pathology are certainly aware of the broad scope that is possible, but believe it is of greater utility to describe healthy narcissism with terms that do not use the word "narcissism." This trend is in accord with the everyday use of narcissism. It also appears to meet a need to have a concept that can be seen in opposition to interest in others, or to altruism, but it is questionable whether having narcissism refer to pathology is of greater utility or clarity than qualifying narcissism as healthy or pathological. Another possibility is to use situational definitions which would shift in their specifics, but that requires a frame of reference, as self-regard, cohesiveness of the self, or libidinal investment, so the specificity and clarity are still attached to a more complex generality.

Reviewing these many attempts to develop an effective definition of narcissism does point out that although perfection is frequently designated as a characteristic of narcissism, perfection is an unlikely result of the pursuit of definition. Given the lack of consensus we are going to have to settle for a relatively acceptable solution. There are common themes that have evolved through the defining process. The first of these is the importance of a notion of the self, even if it remains difficult to define.   The second is the view of an interactional, intersubjective world of the self with objects, self-objects, and self-reflexivity.   These notions are representational in that they exist as mental content and as such have points of reference.   These reference points are personal, namely coming from the individual, and external, namely coming from others.   Narcissism can then be defined as the personal point of reference, or the individual viewpoint whose mental content involves both ideas and affects that have motivational properties. Narcissism can be compared with the viewpoints of others, but personal and external attitudes are potentially interactive rather than exclusive and are subject to each other's influences.

The mental content has rudimentary origins and narcissism begins at whatever moment in life a point of view is formed in the most primitive manner.   This would mean that initially narcissism will be primarily sensory and will be whatever satisfies the needs of the organism at the moment, a primitive unplesaure-pleasure or demand-satisfaction attitude comprised of basic sensations becoming affects, and undoubtedly limited in representational capacity.   Such a point of view is rudimentary yet interactive because of its environmental dependence. The development of a self can be conceptualized as beginning with these sensorimotor experiences that mark the initial stages of life.   From the start there is some form of a personal reference point that motivates the person, and that is the most productive way to describe narcissism.

Maturation of what are generally termed the ego functions will result in an elaboration or structuring of this point of view so that concepts such as self-representations and object-representations become applicable.   The affective, interpersonal, and ideational components of narcissism will be more apparent in motivational sequences of actions and reactions to the self and others.   The developing needs of the individual to survive, adapt, and grow express the personal perspective of narcissism.   This growth often takes place within the context of relationships which foster personal perspectives as well as shaping them to recognize and understand the needs of others and to establish the position of personal needs relative to the needs of others.   In this process, external needs are affected by personal perspectives as the personal and external interact and react to each other.

Narcissism is each person's way of looking at the world and establishing their place within it.   In doing so each person will use whatever mechanisms are available to negotiate their position.   Thus concepts such as autism, symbiosis, merger, fusion, and omnipotence, to whatever extent they may be established as mental mechanisms, can be brought into action in the service of narcissism. However, these ways of relating to the self and others are not necessary for the development of narcissism, and narcissism is not given birth with the formation of a self-representation or through particular libidinal distributions. Instead, narcissism begins when the person begins, and while the concepts mentioned, as well as others described in the review, can be used to describe features of narcissism as it develops or is being expressed, the key feature is the *personal perspective*. This perspective undergoes transformation in service of adaptation, and parental figures clearly play a significant role in this, as does the broader society.

Conflict between one person's narcissism and the narcissism of others is inevitable and provides opportunities for shaping and reshaping one's personal perspective. What is generally described as pathological narcissism represents a range of difficulties in adjusting that perspective. The direction of the adjustment is not predetermined by the presence of conflict. In some instances the person may need to strengthen the existing perspective, while in others the personal perspective will need to be altered. Because conflict is interactive, the perspectives of others can also be changed.

The operation of narcissism can be illustrated through reflexive self-experience. Both subjective self-awareness and objective self-awareness are parts of narcissism as a personal perspective, with conflict appearing in discrepancies between the two modes of self-awareness that are experienced negatively, engendering unpleasant affects such as anxiety, depression, and shame. The person can react to create a less disturbing personal perspective by continually reevaluating both components of awareness so that there will be differing self-perspectives that appear and reappear until alignment occurs. Defense and behavioral alterations are possibilities, but narcissism is the perspective, as compared with being primarily a defensive illusion. Even when the perspective is disturbing, it may be tolerated as still another way to handle the conflict. This means that narcissism is a personal vantage point that seeks an acceptable level of comfort or satisfaction. Sometimes narcissism is very congruent with reality, whereas at other times it sees through distorted lenses and is maladaptive or pathological (Welt & Herron, 1990). In the latter the central feature seems to be an insistence on a personal perspective that essentially lacks the perspective of others and uses defensive measures to avoid recognition or integration of perspectives outside of a fragile preformed one that cannot tolerate changes. Such a picture presents narcissism gone awry, essentially a maladaptive personal perspective that tries to remain frozen rather than to be fluid and adaptive. A crucial distinction needs to be maintained here between disordered narcissism and narcissism as a disorder, because people who display the characteristic of a narcissistic personality disorder are often referred to as "narcissistic," implying that narcissism is to be equated with pathology.

In summary, narcissism is a description of a personal perspective that is naturally self-preservative and self-enhancing through adaptive behaviors that develop within an interactive relational context. Narcissism is designed to assist the individual through the medium of a personally meaningful vantage point for agency and cohesion. As such it operates as a motivational force. The vantage point is also subject to inaccuracies under the influence of negative affects usually engendered by negative parental and societal influences. The pathological adaptations described involve self-image, identity, and relational distortions that reflect a skewed personal perspective.

Narcissism as described is an aspect of major existing developmental conceptions, such as drive, ego, relational, and self. It is more apparent in the latter two as an integral part of the structuring process for development of the self and of object relations because these clearly involve a personal perspective. The influence of narcissism is also seen in drive expression and the use of ego functions such as judgement and reality testing, and particularly in adaptation. The proposed definition avoids being restrictive and does not rely on only a particular psychoanalytic school of thought, but by using the term "personal perspective" it requires a developmental schema for the person or the self. This feature will be considered in more detail in the next chapter as we examine narcissistic motivation in personality development.

II
The Development of Narcissism

In the first chapter I proposed a working definition of narcissism as the personal perspective, or individual point of view. This perspective is composed of cognitive and affective elements that combine to produce a personal motivational attitude that is reflected in each person's behavior. The terms *personal*, *individual*, and *person* have as their referent the construct of *self*, which will be amplified in this chapter. The terms *perspective*, *point of view*, and *motivational attitude* are the developmental components of narcissism that originate in sensorimotor patterns that mature into cognitive-affective schemata. We will begin with a discussion of the many possible definitions of the self, and follow that with a depiction of narcissism as a major motivational force.

The Self

When Hartmann (1950) shifted the target of narcissism from the ego to the self he kept the self as a component of the ego, as did Jacobson (1964), and the self became equivalent to an image, or representation of the self, as distinguished from an object-representation. Grey (1993a) has suggested that the term "self" is customarily reserved for social transactions, so that the self is viewed in the context of relationships, the "I" as distinct from the "you," or "other," and that the self is the person as an object of reflective consciousness, namely aware of and evaluating oneself. Grey then suggests two major differing perspectives of the self, endogenous and interactional.

The endogenous perspective emphasizes a developmental pattern for an entity with specific characteristics, such as autonomy and consistency, whereas the interactional position views the self as a personal construct with varying characteristics. The degree of interaction with interpersonal contexts, and their influence, are the primary distinctions. For example, Jacobson described self -representations as "unconscious, preconscious, and conscious endopsychic representations of the bodily, and mental self in the system ego" (1964, p.16). The self is subjective experience, that depending on the perspective, was more (interactional) or less (endogenous) subject to environmental influences.

The evolution of psychoanalytic theory has elaborated the self as primarily an interactional construct. Individuals are viewed as social participants who through experience with others develop observational standpoints that guide attention, perception, and role development (Grey, 1993a). These guiding observational standpoints are congruent with the definition of narcissism as a personal perspective.

The interactive view begins with Sullivan (1954) and the description of the self-system as processes, states, symbols, and signs functioning to primarily provide security. This self-system included the personified self, which is the self of which one is aware. Grey (1993b) suggests that there is an ongoing exchange between a subjective world and external interactions that rules out a private self that is unaffected by others, just as social interactions must be affected by subjectivity. However, the continuity of interaction is less demonstrable than the presence of an interaction, so the degree of interaction, and in turn the relativity of the "untouched" nature of the self remains a question. In this vein, consider Winnicott's (1965) interest in the privacy of subjectivity and the personal, isolated core self.

Grey (1993b) describes the self as containing self-reflexive skills and knowledge, and being a personalized part of a self-system. This system uses unaware assessments for continuous reorganization and coordination with personality resources to cope with ongoing situations. Both conscious and unconscious aspects of the self-system are viewed as intuitively attuned to the self as integrating or coping tendencies. The primary motivational affects and needs are found in relationships that influence self-esteem, particularly the quality of approval and disapproval coming from significant others.

The self of self-psychology appears less relational due to its emphasis on the nuclear self, but Fosshage (1992) suggests that due to self-experience developing in a relational matrix, self-psychology is basically a relational model, a view that is reinforced by the concept of intersubjectivity (Atwood & Stolorow, 1984) that emphasizes the interaction of subjectivities. The definition of the self is not precise. Instead, emphasis is given to its experiential aspects, such as "center of activity," "independent center of initiative," and "intrinsic program of action." Although self-psychology emphasizes experience rather than structure (Lichtenberg, 1991), there is a structural notion of a core self that tends to be present in most descriptions of the self. The self is also considered to have an inherent developmental program, but one that requires relationships (Fosshage, 1992). Self-development contains the motivation to achieve self-cohesion, and maintain it, through self-selfobject relationships, but tilts towards viewing others as facilitating objects without mutual recognition of subject and objects (Benjamin, 1992).

Mitchell (1992) prefers to view the self as a temporal concept, namely the subjective organization of meanings created as a person moves in time. The emphasis is on experience, with a distinction between authenticity and inauthenticity based more on the relationship between feeling and action than the content of feelings and actions. However, it is possible to retain the spatial metaphor and add the temporal, experiential dimension. For example, the self has been described as a center for motivation, with a sense of self coming from experiencing the motivational activity (Lichtenberg, 1989). Modell (1994) stresses the idea of a private self with an inner core that is in opposition to environmental impingements. Thus, the description by Winnicott of an environmental situation where the individual "exists by not being found" (1958, p.212).

Pine (1990) describes the psychology of self-experience, considering the self as an experiential construct and the individual in terms of ongoing subjective states. The states specified are boundaries, authenticity, agency, and affective tone. Boundaries refer to the degree of self-differentiation and separateness. Authenticity is seen in the context of the true and false self distinction. Agency is the individual's sense of being able to live life as an active agent, and affective tone is concerned with wholeness, continuity, and self-esteem. An emphasis is given to self-definition in relation to others. The subjective states are essentially motivational in that there are ongoing efforts to maintain a comfortable and familiar subjective sense of self.

This overview of perspectives on the self indicates agreement as to the existence and importance of the self, as well as an increased emphasis on subjective experience and the development of subjective states in relation to others, but the concept remains difficult to define. The subjective "I" as experience rather than an entity has considerable support based on the possible limitations of a spatial metaphor, namely that it emphasizes a one-person psychology with the person as a closed system and that it reifies the construct rather than retaining the metaphorical tone that was intended (Lichtenberg, Lachmann, & Fosshage, 1992). However, the metaphorical use of a spatial description has the attractions of historical precedence, convenience, and illustrative evocation. For example, in attempting to operationalize the self-representation, Bocknek and Perona (1994) note that body image is an obvious representation of the self and reflects meaning about the self. A spatial description of the self gives a tangible, pictorial flavor to the experiences that are the domain of an entity that is having the mental and physical experiences. There is an experiencing self that can be reflective and descriptive, and there is an experienced self that constitutes accessible past activity no longer being experienced, and in turn an unconscious experiencing self as well as an unconscious experienced self that are essentially out-of-awareness potentials that may or may not become available for reflective mental experience. Because of the comprehensive nature of the self it then is accurate to view the self as the person, and to describe its aspects separately, as experiencing self, self-representation, etc. The self manifests itself to an individual and to others as some type of representation, at times sensory, at times perceptual, as well as in combination.

The experience of the self translates into who I am, who I appear to be, who I imagine myself to be, as well as the thinking, feeling, perceiving, reflecting person. Self-representation is a central feature, as noted by Sandler (1986), in reflecting on the original descriptions of the self by Hartmann and Jacobson, and is interconnected with object representations, but the self does not have to be categorized as part of the ego. Shane and Shane (1980) consider the options of locating the self within the psychic apparatus or within the person, and prefer the latter. The self as self-representation appears less viable than the broader construct of the self as the entire person. A position akin to this, although stressing self-experience, is the depiction of the self as a superordinate concept, namely "an independent center for initiating, organizing, and integrating experience and motivation" (Lichtenberg, et al., 1992, p.58).

Narcissism then is a basic part of the self, the perspective of the person that in turn plays a major motivational role in all human behavior. This is apparent in what Mitchell (1992) describes as the dialectic between self-expression and interpersonal security and in what Benjamin (1992) depicts as the tension between recognizing the other and asserting the self. These are essentially adaptive situations, fundamental to the process of relating, which illustrate how the narcissism of one person interacts with the narcissism of another, or others, and motivates behavior. Lichtenberg et al. (1992) have proposed a framework for mental activity that illustrates the possibilities for narcissism, namely the intrapsychic, the intersubjective, and self-states. The intrapsychic includes responses to the person's different priorities of motivation, whereas the intersubjective refers to responses to the experienced needs of others, and the self-state is the affective-cognitive-kinesthetic self-organization that affects and reflects the intrapsychic and the intersubjective. Such self-organization is both the result and determiner of narcissism. The next sections will explore the developmental patterns of narcissism as a personal perspective and the activation of its motivational force.

Personal Perspectives

Narcissism is a basic motivational construct that describes the need to service the self in accord with ongoing evaluations of the requirements for self-satisfaction. Part of the need is met almost automatically, with little thought. Many bodily functions exemplify this, such as breathing. More of the need, however, has to do with goals that require thought, where decisions are made on the basis of cognition and emotion that specific behavior is of value. Some of this is relatively automatic, but based on past experience and subject to correction if current experience proves negative. For example, driving the same route to work based on its brevity, but altering it if traffic patterns result in delays not previously experienced. Social relations can also have primarily automatic patterns as well, but these are learned over time as the best ways for a person to operate in given situations. These patterns are also subject to change if they are ineffective, but their ineffectiveness is often less apparent to a person because the patterns themselves provide satisfactions that are not easily replaced, or because the qualities of other people may be seen as the cause of the difficulty. In both cases the person acts in a set way because the person continues to believe that it is better than trying a different way. Of course behavior that is clearly effective will be reinforcing, so the motivation is apparent. In all cases, however, the judgement as to the value of behavior rests on a personal perspective, namely, doing what appears to be good for the self.

The personal perspective begins when the person begins, but is not formalized as a representational process until the cognitive and affective components have matured sufficiently to permit self-representations and object-representation. However, it is important to recognize that the individual is striving from conception to satisfy personal needs. The natural tendency of the organism is to grow using available resources. This growth appears to be initially recognized by others before it is recognized by the person, yet there is always some internal sense that there is a developing person. This development has a guiding principle, a sense of "what to do" that could also be described as narcissism, and that is continually influenced by the narcissism of others.

During development a person is also subject to internal and external misguiding. Some of this occurs because of a lack of knowledge about the results of action, as when a child hurts herself in an exploratory activity such as touching a hot surface. Some occurs because of trust in others who have provided erroneous directions, often unintentionally. For example, a parent may urge a child to try to do something without realizing the child is not yet emotionally prepared and therefore is destined to fail. Also, misguiding may occur when people believe they are acting in their own best interests, but they are not. This type of miscalculation is essentially the result of defensive affects which prevent a recognition of the most likely result, or of events that could not be anticipated. However, in these instances people feel they are being true to their narcissism. For example, anxiety about communicating with another person can mask the necessity of communication in a particular situation. The person believes it is better to cater to the anxiety than to speak when he is anxious, but he turns out to be incorrect. A similar problem can occur when action is delayed in the belief that there will be another, better opportunity, but there is not.

Although it is probable that infants have an early narcissism that is primarily informative coming from proprioceptive and somatosensory sources, and have the capacity to organize experience in an adaptive manner, the narcissism is immature and error prone. Thus, even with the maturation of experience and the central nervous system, the self remains vulnerable to both the effects of narcissistic injuries as they occur and to their lingering effects. Maturing narcissism remains error prone as it is difficult to truly serve the self. The problem of being in one's most satisfying narcissistic state is illustrated by the following clinical example.

A female patient tells her male therapist, "You are going to laugh at this, but I sometimes think of myself as a lethal weapon."

He laughs because in their therapy up to this point both of them have experienced her as the overly willing recipient of others' aggression. Her narcissism has been reflected in her role as a container of hostile familial emotions. She has been afraid to either fight back or assert herself, and she prefers the role of victim to being the victimizer, which is her perception of herself in any role but being the victim. He also interprets the "lethal weapon" to be the result of her built up rage, her identification with the aggressor, her desire to be a way that she also fears.

She agrees, chides him for laughing at her, being the aggressor, having set him up to laugh so that the image could be tempered a bit. Yet she is also sad. She states that she is "very sad," but lapses into "I don't know" when asked about her sadness.

The therapist wonders, what if he had not laughed? What if he had taken the "lethal weapon" seriously? What had she wanted, and now, what next?

In this segment, the patient's narcissism keeps shifting, at least in terms of what is apparent. She wants a response from the therapist, but offers choices to him without giving him a clear direction. He responds in a way that has been familiar to both of them, an acknowledgment and sharing of her masochistic dependency, which is also a type of maternal omnipotence in her ability to calmly contain everyone's aggression. However, she is not comfortable with his response.

She presented at least two possibilities, a sharing of amusement or a sharing of concern at her rage. It appears that she was more interested in the latter, but when the therapist shifts in that direction she becomes sad and distant. There are of course other ways that the therapist could have responded, including just listening, but regardless of the response, the patient's perspective is difficult to discern. How is she serving herself when she presents herself as the "lethal weapon?" What is known to her about her motivation and what is unknown? Does she have a particular goal in mind that is actually pursued throughout, such as discomforting the therapist, or being unable to get solace, or is she ambivalent and changing goals? These are all possibilities, and there are undoubtedly other possibilities. The woman's perspective is a mixture of conscious and unconscious motivation so that it is partially aware and deliberate as well as automatic, unaware, and uncertain. There is nonetheless a narcissistic perspective that could be determined, perhaps in a continued dialogue between the patient and the therapist, or through self-reflection, or through both. It is this perspective that is the "guiding hand" for the way she presents, the story she tells, and the way she tells it. An understanding of the patient for herself and for the therapist rests upon discovering her narcissism.

For example, she may feel sad because she has been stimulated to have that feeling as a way to express a need, which in this case can be assumed to be a mixture of needing to discharge the feeling, to have it register to herself to impel and validate activity or passivity, and to have the therapist react to her. At the same time, other needs may appear, such as regret at the way she is now depicting herself, or anger that her anger is being blunted by the sadness, so that as she moves into this state of sadness she is also in conflict and wishes for a different state, namely the return of the "lethal weapon."

Thus the personal perspective is frequently a shifting one as the person struggles to find a way to be that best expresses the narcissism that exists in contexts of both conflict, as competing needs, and deficit, as a lack of sources of satisfaction. This struggle is a developmental process that will be lifelong and therefore only relatively successful given the oppositional qualities of both drives and relations. However, the degree of success can be sufficiently satisfying that people are both motivated to seek it and do enjoy a sense of completeness for significant periods of time. Thus narcissism involves continually developing and perceiving a personal perspective with the goal of gratification, as well as being able to accept disappointment, tolerate frustration, and delay satisfaction.

Developmental Processes

Body signals are the first sign of narcissism. The body-self attempts to get satisfaction through both tension reduction and stimulation. In so doing there is a beginning of a supply of experience that is used by the self to learn its needs and how they can be satisfied. At the same time, signals are sent to caretakers that demands are being made, and their acknowledgement of the narcissism interactively shapes its development.

Major developmental schema are useful for understanding the direction of narcissism. For example, in the first year of life oral satisfaction is a major concern, so that feeding patterns can be thought of in terms of their timing and style. They reflect what the infant wants, and what the parents want, and how desires meet and reach a settlement. Also, normal autism, normal symbiosis, and the beginning of separation-individuation have been proposed for this time period (Mahler, Pine, & Bergman, 1975). Although the phase-dominance of autism in particular has not been supported, it is useful to note the presence of stimulus avoidance along with stimulus-seeking. The holding environment described by Winnicott (1965) illustrates the cyclical experience of formless quiescence and active demands by the infant. The issue of symbiosis is also intriguing because Hofer (1994) has argued from biological evidence that even when infants could survive on their own they give a portion of control of their internal environment to their mothers, and that there is a dual unity of homeostatic systems that makes symbiosis an appropriate term. The sharing of functions of course does not rule out differentiation and is not equivalent to the absence of separate selves. Some type of symbiosis appears in concepts such as mutual cueing, the mother-infant unit, the object as an auxiliary ego, and mutual influence (Beebe & Lachman, 1992). These concepts are similar in their emphasis on mutuality while they differ in the degree to which they see the partners in the dyad as capable of recognizing each other. For example, symbiosis as originally proposed provides for limited external awareness and emphasizes merging, whereas mutual influence supports the representational capacity of the infant from birth.

The first year of life represents an interaction between the infant and other people that illustrates both togetherness and separateness. The most frequent progression described has been from extreme togetherness to separation and individuation that will include mutuality, although Stern (1985) has raised questions about this sequence. It is not necessary, however, to agree on the sequence in order to note that separateness and togetherness are features of a person's life that are of significance from the start. Thus part of narcissism is the desire for separateness, togetherness, aloneness, and mutuality. The description of the separation-individuation phase observed in the first year of life, namely hatching and practicing, are useful in understanding the dyadic model.

Also useful are the stages of self-experience and social relatedness described by Stern (1985). For the first years of life these are the emergent self, the core self, and the beginning of the subjective self at about seven months. These senses of the self are described as subjective perspectives that organize experience, and therefore fit a motivational view of narcissism. The emergent self refers to both the process and the results of forming relations between separate experiences. It is an experience of organization beginning with the body. The core self builds upon the emergent self to develop the four senses of agency, coherence, affectivity, and continuity, as organized experiences. The *sense* of self is emphasized to highlight experience in contrast to the core self as a cognitive construct, but to describe a sense of self as an experiential integration still seems to be depicting a construct because it requires conceptualization to understand it, and it is reasonable to assume that varying degrees of comprehension accompany the experience, particularly the organization of experiences. The central theme of organization with intentionality fits well with the perspective of narcissism.

It is not necessary to subscribe to a particular belief in the primacy of a domain of experience, as drives or relations, to utilize the observations of different models as contributors to the development of narcissism. Although it is accurate to note that contemporary psychoanalytic theory and practice favors addressing relational motivation and its products, the primacy of any model, as well as the integration of models, remain as controversial issues. The personal perspective exists regardless of the outcome of these controversies, and their ingredients provide information about narcissism.

We have focused upon Freud's psychosexual model, Mahler's relational model, and Stern's model of self-development, but other models are also useful contributors to narcissistic content and style. To mention just a few, there are the organizer's of the psyche (Spitz, 1959), starting with the smiling response in the first year, followed by stranger anxiety and the "No" response. This model has been elaborated by Tyson and Tyson (1990) in a blend with stages of cognitive integration (Piaget & Inhelder, 1969) and the developmental lines proposed by Anna Freud (1965) into a broad theory of development with a number of evolving, interdependent systems.

Another example is the developmental structuralist model (Greenspan, 1990) which emphasizes stage-tasks and capacities beginning with homeostasis. Also included within the first year are attachment, somatopsychological differentiation, and the beginning of behavioral organization. All these models have an emphasis and are more or less integrative, and are selective in data interpretation, yet in their respective points of view illustrate that narcissism has a lot of areas for expression. Thus, at any given moment a person's narcissism may reflect, in varying degrees, drives, structures, affects, cognitions, relations, and values in a particular, subjective way.

During the first year of life the use of the body, relations to others, and cognitive and emotional awareness have been emphasized by developmental theorists. The principal disputes have been about the degree to which the developing child is aware of the self and of others, and the degree to which the self is differentiated from others through the formation of self-representations and object-representations, as well as whether there is a dominant need to have contact with others, or whether the major motivation is the expression of drives such as libido and aggression through the mechanism of others. For example, is attachment a motivation distinct from libidinal expression (Bowlby, 1969) or is it an expression of the libidinal drive?

The current direction of psychoanalytic developmental theory favors considerable awareness by the infant at birth and considerable interest in others to the point that early undifferentiation and drive dominance are called into question. At the same time cognitive and affective processes do undergo maturation, body-based urges are powerful motives, and the need for relatedness is not necessarily the major motivational force. It does seem, given the increasing evidence as to the abilities and capacities of the infant from birth, or even from conception, that there is from the start an endowed person who makes use of the environment to develop capacities. There appears to be some type of perceptual interactive organization for the person which emphasizes growth and development for all of the characteristics of the person. This organization is facilitated by maturation, drive presence, and interpersonal experience. The use of facilitators is governed by narcissism with decisions by the person to act in a particular way, as in the beginning to cry, and later, to speak. The cognitive reflective aspect of the decision of course is increased with central nervous system development as well as with experience. If the self is viewed as the total person, then the person is always seeking to do something that the self will experience positively, and there are always evaluations followed by decisions as to what action will take place.

Providing an explanation for the advent of self-reflexive awareness has always been an issue for psychoanalytic theorists. Many theorists who emphasize the limits of awareness in the first year of life based on the need for maturation also include concepts that seem to involve representational thought, such as hallucinatory wishes and infantile omnipotence, that are not congruent with the maturational capacities of the infant. The same problem occurs with some theories that increase the level of differentiation of self and others, such as the work of Melanie Klein (1952) which accelerates the conceptual aspects of relationships beyond the realities of age-determined cognition. Both drive theorists and relational theorists do this. As an example of the latter, Winnicott proposes infant hallucination and hallucinatory omnipotence. In apparent contrast, Greenspan (1990) delays the representational capacity until the second year of life, although he believes there is an earlier capacity to organize experience. Stern (1985) has noted that some theorists contend symbolic functions are too limited prior to 12 months to consider self-awareness a meaningful attribute, and others see 18 to 24 months as the dividing line. Clearly there is disagreement as to the point of entry for motivational organization that can be considered indicative of a self.

However, all theories seem to agree that there is a motivational organization, and it is useful to have concepts that describe the organization in categorical terms, such as the classic triad of id, ego, and superego, or the self, that are viewed as metaphorical mental structures for functions and experiences. Recent evidence supports the existence of the self at birth, with limited self-reflection and representational power. In the first years of life there are signs of an early representational system that precedes symbolic functioning (Beebe & Lachmann, 1992). Such a presymbolic representational capacity, along with evidence of patterns of interactive infant-caretaker regulation, provide a basis for symbolic self- and object representations. They also support the existence of a self at birth, described by Stern (1985) as the sense of an emergent self. Wolf (1980) also notes that caretakers imagine the neonate to have a self, which Kohut termed the virtual self, and this is communicated to the infant who does appear to respond to it. Although Wolf is cautious about the degree of organization of the self at birth, the sense of an emerging self seems quite appropriate. Furthermore, Stern notes that infants seek stimulation, have preferences, and are constantly evaluating the similarities and differences of experience. This evaluative process corresponds to the proposed conception of narcissism in that it is part of the decision making that leads to the furthering of the self-interest. The facilitators of narcissism in the first year of life are bodily-based, such as drive discharges and sensory stimulation, and outside the self, primarily the activity of caretakers. The facilitators are interactive, establishing a model that continues through the life span. Descriptions of the activities of this time span, and corresponding models, are guides to the details for narcissistic development.

The second year of life emphasizes the clash of wills between parents and the child in the anal period, as well as the discovery of the joys and risks of separation-individuation in the practicing and rapprochement subphases. The senses of the self emphasize subjectivity and the beginnings of a verbal self. Physical and sensory differentiation of the self and others provide a foundation for an intersubjective relatedness. Self- and object representations are generally considered to be in place, and there is a desire to share experiences with others, to be known as well as to know others, particularly in terms of feelings.

It is more apparent to the person in this time period than in the first year that gratification and satisfaction require cooperation with others. There are precursors to this awareness in the oral period, despite depictions such as infantile omnipotence, because the infant is extremely dependent and must develop ways to get others to be good caretakers. It is true that mothers are often particularly motivated, and that less is expected of the infant than the two year old. However, patterns of infant-caretaker mutual regulation are being created from birth and constitute presymbolic representations. These involve expectancies of both regulation and misregulation, which although considered interactive with a simultaneous structuring of self and object experiences (Beebe & Lechmann, 1992), involve processes of reciprocal adjustment. Thus, the infant is not omnipotent, but has to adjust to the mother just as she has to adjust to the infant. The mother tends to be more willing to try to meet apparent demands in the first year without being demanding, but it is a reciprocal process with the infant learning what to do to get demands met, and that learning is the development of a personal perspective that goes beyond bodily responses.

Lichtenberg et al. (1992) have described the development from birth of motivational systems that include self-organization, self-stabilization, dialectic tension, and hierarchical arrangement. For example, environmental exploration appears as the result of the motivation to organize. In the beginning there is feedback contingent awareness accompanied by interest in reexperiencing activities. In addition to physiological and attachment satisfactions there are perceptual activity and interest patterns as well as the development of efficiency and competence, both of which being developmental tasks that are primary in the second year in relation to parental approval regarding delay and control.

Internal regulation and external regulation have their start in the first year and are prominent in the second year. In addition, there can be a conflict at any point of maturational transition between the former familiar mode of existence and a new, unfamiliar type of experience. All instances illustrate preferences and choices that become the content of narcissism. There are innate preferences for sensory modalities, such as for auditory, visual or tactile processing, as well as for types of stimuli and the manner of stimulus presentation. Then there are choices to be made in terms of actions that involve or require others, with mutual communication well before the advent of verbalization.

Lichtenberg (1983) suggests that at about nine months the imaging capacity is developed. This has been preceded by recognition, but this is qualified by the object and the action being connected so that the object is not yet independent. As the imagery capacity develops the self and object begin to develop a separate existence with the representation subsequently being in word symbols. The second organizer of the psyche, stranger anxiety, is suggested at about nine months. When this is apparent it appears to be a reaction to people whose affect state cannot be readily understood. This is a reflection of the development of the affective exchanges that have been taking place between the child and caretakers. These affective signposts are further indications of subjective preferences.

In the second year conflicts occur between toddlers and parents that have been attributed to a variety of sources such as retention-expulsion, rapprochement, and different methods of processing information. These struggles illustrate the will of the child as it shapes others and is being shaped by others. Lichtenberg et al. (1992) emphasize the changes that occur in cognition, perception, and problem solving that are underscored by the myelination of associational pathways. There appears to be a hierarchical arrangement of motivations that reflects choices and intentionality influenced by both conscious and unconscious factors to different degrees in each person. Developmental stage theories generally support such a hierarchical arrangement, with an emphasis on a growing sense of competency that can be viewed as a firming up of narcissism.

Lichtenberg (1983) illustrates the growth of preferential dominance in regard to cognitive control where individual differences can be categorized as alternative modes of exploration. Cognitive styles are established, such as low or high scanning (the degree to which attention is directed toward the external world), field-articulation, tolerance of unreality, and leveling or sharpening. These cognitive styles can be viewed as examples of narcissistic styles where each tendency is essentially a preferred choice. This appears congruent with Stern's (1985) conception of early presymbolic representations that reflect central experiential elements of motivational systems. Life begins with organizing and integrating capacities that are the origins of narcissism as a subjective perspective that forms and reforms within an interpersonal context.

The personal perspective that is narcissism will be reflected throughout life. I have focused on its early development to make the point that narcissism is an originating concept that is relatively well formed as a motivational force during the second year of life. The further development of narcissism will now be described in the Oedipal period which starts with the third year of life, a point at which object constancy is also thought to be significantly on its way to being established. Object constancy also refers to self-constancy, or the viewing of the self as both a congruent subject and object. Constancy highlights the ability to look at both the self and others and form evaluations that lead to affective and cognitive conclusions. In particular it becomes possible to categorize people as good or bad, likeable or not likeable, in relative terms rather than absolute dichotomies. Temporal variations are also possible to allow for changes of feeling and perception, and varying degrees of ambivalence are expected. In essence, a relative view of self and others develops that allows for the retention of impressions over time and without the presence of the other person. The self and other are also viewed as having mixtures of qualities yet permitting dominant impressions to be formed on one or the other side of the ambivalence, and with gradations of attraction. This is a complex view, in that the impression that is formed can be relatively constant despite actual changes in the object, as well as fluctuating due to changes in the subject. In that view object constancy could be seen as primarily a function of personal impressions of the value of the object to the subject, with changes in perspective, or an inflexibility of perspective being based on how the person needs to perceive the object. The object world is therefore organized by the person to provide consistency and stability, and to facilitate interpersonal exchanges which are also aided by the development of the verbal self and a variety of cognitive and affective ego functions.

The Oedipal period is usually thought of as a time when gender identity, sexual preference, and object choice are established. Two major processes occur, identification and libidinal object choice. The normal pattern is male identification and female object choice, or female identification and male object choice, with a correspondence between biological maleness or femaleness and psychological male and female identity. However, the psychological identities do not have to correspond to appropriate-sex libidinal preferences, so both homosexuality and bisexuality are possibilities. In addition, although there are qualities that are often considered to be masculine or feminine, these are not essential to a male or female identity, instead being determined more by societal expectations and functional expectancies.

At issue for understanding narcissism is the question of choice in regard to the characteristics of a person's identity. The psychosexual stages emphasize a biological, phallocentric base which through a combination of fear and positive identification result in heterosexual identity as a normal developmental pattern. Other models have subsequently been proposed (Fast, 1984; Stoller, 1985) that make use of more recent data to support a greater emphasis on learning, the role of society, and the separate task of boys and girls in becoming men and women.

As the mother is the first contact object and the early caretaker, the early identification and libidinal preferences are for her, although the designation of boy or girl is made by the parents to the child. This gender designation is then reinforced by the attitudes of others, so that a girl's identification with her mother would receive external support, while the boy would be shifted toward the father by others. In addition, to the degree that the child is aware of it, anatomical similarities and differences would support the biological gender identity. Awareness of their genitals and the anatomical differences between the sexes appears to occur for both boys and girls between 14 and 24 months (Riophe & Galenson, 1981).The awareness of a designated boy or girl identity of course has preceded the knowledge of what that means functionally, so a sorting out process continues in terms of understanding the male and female roles. A variety of intense emotions, as love, hatred, envy, and fear, accompany the process and affect it.

There are a number of points at which important individual perspectives are developed. Anatomy has supplied one agent of destiny, but there are choices in the specifics of being a male and being a female, and within the broad categories of heterosexual and homosexual there is considerable variation in intensity, style, and consequence. Also, it is common to identify with characteristics of each parent despite having a singular gender identity, and the particulars of male and female roles in the society are open to variations. Concepts such as penis envy and castration anxiety can be seen as ways in which the child is evaluating identities.

For the boy, the developmental tasks appears to be the establishment of a male identity and a corresponding libidinal object choice. These tasks involve making an identity shift from the mother to the father, and a libidinal shift from the mother to an age-appropriate non-familial female. The initial identity appears to be a contact identity, both physical and psychological, and the identity of familiar person recognition. There seems to be a wish to be like the gratifier, or in case the gratification is insufficient or absent, to incorporate what one can of who is available and known, and libidinal feeling is also likely to go more easily to the initial object. The boy is presented with the task of being interested in the mother as the model of a woman, without becoming himself the woman-mother, yet with considerable room for being like the mother, with society providing cues as to how to accomplish this, along with the mother and father teaching their own views of what a boy and a man are to be. The girl can solidify her initial identification with the mother, but is expected as a key part of her feminine identity to move her libidinal interests to the father as the model for her subsequent opposite-sex preference. Of course she will identify with aspects of the father that appeal to her, but is expected to retain and further a primary identification with a female, maternal role.

It is quite possible that role developments away from these norms represent apparently adaptive choices that are partially influenced by biological-genetic components. The issue of the causes of sexual preferences remains unsettled (Bleckner, 1995, 1996; Herron & Herron, 1995; Tabin, 1995,1996), particularly in terms of the roles of heredity and environment in creating libidinal preferences, but the involvement of narcissism is apparent in that there is a desire to gratify the self through getting one's preference. The likeness of the object to the self, which is superficially apparent in homosexuality, is no more narcissistic however than the choice of a sexual object of the opposite sex based on an identity of personal characteristics. If these are essentially merger situations, then they may reflect pathological narcissism. In contrast, the progression of normal, healthy narcissism requires an investment in the subjectivity of others in order to facilitate personal adaptation. The personal perspective is within the interpersonal field, so that one looks out for the self by looking out for others who are a part of a reciprocal loop from which all parties draw psychological satisfaction. This point has been made in different terms by Benjamin (1992) in her exploration of learning to see the other as a subject, and by self psychology in considering how the self learns the value of being a selfobject. It is applicable to heterosexuality, homosexuality, and bisexuality.

Also, narcissism is involved in another aspect of identification, namely the internalization of values on a selective basis to form the superego as part of the resolution of the Oedipal conflicts that result in the appropriate shaping of desire. In psychosexual models the superego has precursors, and perhaps a preoedipal formation in relational models. Self psychology gives idealization and the development of ambitions and goals a basic role in the bipolar self (Lee & Martin, 1991) that is congruent with narcissism as the personal perspective.

Gottschalk (1990) traces the course of narcissism through the life cycle, distinguishing between healthy and pathological narcissism. He notes that there are challenges to narcissism from birth to age five that can aid acculturation and the sense of reality. At the same time, rejecting or exploiting parents can contribute to a distorted sense of entitlement, as can overly indulgent parents. From five to ten societal standards are seen as major vehicles for developing self-esteem. This is further emphasized in adolescence with needs to understand peer groups, sexual roles, and vocational possibilities. The establishment of belief systems, adolescent identity, and the complexity of love relationships all require personal perspectives. In early and middle adulthood developmental tasks that have major narcissistic components include vocational choices, intimate, lasting relations, and a position within the community as well as parental roles. Later adulthood brings still other challenges, such as providing significant economic support for others, coping with retirement, and adapting to physical and mental limitations, as well as to the loss of significant others.

Throughout the life cycle there is movement from relatively unconditional love to more conditional gratification that requires a shifting narcissism that retains and structures the components of the self in a personally adaptive way. Pathological narcissism is essentially depicted by Gottschalk as distortions in self-love and self-respect that appear in many forms of psychopathology, such as depression, rather than just in a narcissistic personality disorder. As for healthy narcissism over time relative to repeated narcissistic injuries, Gottschalk states, "the poor in self-love get poorer and the rich in self-love get richer" (1990, p.77).

Pathological Narcissism

The previous chapter described one trend to restrict the meaning of narcissism to pathology, and described the various characteristics that have been designated as narcissistic personality disorders. However, my perspective is that narcissistic pathology is only one category of narcissism, the other being healthy or normal narcissism, and that pathological narcissism is essentially a maladaptive personal perspective. As such it appears in both the narcissistic personality disorders as well as in other disorders that have signs or symptoms representing subjective distortions. In that sense, narcissism is probably implicated in most mental disorders, and the personal perspective is always something to consider in attempting to understand and treat any disorder, including physical disorders.

The previous focus was on the contribution of narcissistic pathology to the clarification of the meaning of narcissism. At this point the interest is in why certain aspects of narcissism tend to be considered pathological and how these maladaptations are developed. In that context, consideration will be given to the theories of Kernberg (1975), Kohut (1971a, 1971b), Auerbach (1993), Fiscalini (1993), and Bach (1985).

Kernberg utilizes a mixture of drive, structural, and relational concepts to describe a spectrum of narcissism from normal to pathological. He has an affect-driven theory in which feelings are the major organizer of internalized object relations and of motivational drive systems. Thus, although Kernberg describes narcissism as a self-cathexis, the cathexis is affective. In its origin there is a reflection of subjective gratification or frustration of physiological needs. This shifts through developmental stages to become more an encompassing subjective interpretation of the meaning of the affects for both self and other as evaluated through structures such as the ego and the superego. Narcissism is dependent on the development of affects, drives, relations, and structures. This means that narcissism involves the relationships of self and object representations as well as libido and aggression. These representations develop from an undifferentiated self-object representation that is the source of both narcissism and object cathexis. Narcissism and object involvement are complimentary rather than oppositional in their origins and in normal development.

Pathological narcissism develops when oral frustration is created by parents to the point that the infant feels intensely hostile, including resentment, envy, and hatred. As a defensive maneuver there is a fusion of the ideal self, the ideal object, and real self-images, as well as a devaluation and destruction of both object images and objects. Identification with ideal images eliminates the need for depending on external objects. Discrepancies between real and ideal selves are also eliminated through an inflated self-concept, with any unacceptable aspects repressed and projected into devalued objects. Both normal differentiation between ideal self and object images and normal superego are disrupted. Thus the narcissistic perspective is to protect the self from feared others by not needing them, or using them and then discarding them. At the same time, however, the intense rage must be concealed, so there is often an apparent superficial adaptation that is essentially exploitative. The etiology seems to lie in parental failures to provide sufficient narcissistic supplies that may well be coupled with a constitutional predisposition to intense rage which is the predominant reaction to the early deprivation.

Grandiosity, self-absorption, lack of empathy, and the projection of rage are notable characteristics along with feelings of inferiority and insecurity. Defense mechanisms are viewed as similar to a borderline personality organization and include splitting, denial, projective identification, omnipotence, and idealization. The significant others are viewed as strong and containing needed gratification yet not giving, malevolent and threatening, so that experienced rage cannot be expressed toward them, nor can they be depended upon. Splitting permits a shifting categorical perception that avoids ambivalence and restricts anxiety, but diffuses identity. Idealization aids the containment of hostility, as does projective identification, which also facilitates the blurring of boundaries between the self and others. Omnipotence facilitates the feeling of invulnerability. The major dynamic appears to be the erection of defenses against the expression of rage toward pathological internal objects that is primarily a result of intense oral deprivation.

Kohut begins with narcissism as the libidinal cathexis of the self, but is really describing an experiencing of the self with the inclusion of others as selfobjects rather than a quantitative concept of cathexis. Narcissism is seen as a normal developmental process which involves differentiating the self from others through the formation of a bipolar self that contains the grandiose and idealized selves. The developing person has two major needs, namely positive attention from others and opportunities for indulging others. Narcissistic pathology comes about in reaction to parental failures in providing the necessary experiences for the person to develop adequate self-esteem and ideals. Akin to Kernberg, the damage is done in the preoedipal period and occurs through parental failure. The etiology lies in the developmental arrest of progressive growth through interpersonal transactions. Kohut concurs with the picture of excessive grandiosity and self-absorption as narcissistic disorders, but does not see these narcissistic disturbances as arising as a defense against oral rage. Instead the disturbance takes the form of trying to fill in the missing self-object experiences through inappropriate creation of mirroring, merging, and idealizing interactions with others. Rage is seen as a possible reaction to failures in the perfection of the idealized self-object or in the omnipotence of the grandiose self. It is particularly apparent in a lack of empathy, but it is not the key feature of narcissistic disorders. The distorted personal perspective is exhibitionism, grandiosity, and merger that justify rage, exaggerated personal claims, and the desire for control and omnipotence at the expense of others. Pathological narcissism is considered archaic, or untransformed narcissism. Then grandiosity appears as unrealistic expectations of the self, shame, self-criticism, attempts at absolute control, and excessive longing for connections to idealized others. This is essentially a "softer" picture of pathological narcissism because it gives less emphasis to aggression than the depiction by Kernberg, although it is clear that the transferences of the narcissistic person described by Kohut, as idealizing, mirroring, and twinship, have significant aggressive features in their expectations of the analyst. Kernberg's narcissists seem to be trying to find an appropriate way to express aggression, whereas Kohut's narcissists appear to be looking to fill an experiential void. Both groups need others, but in their personal perspectives, narrow their focus to a self-absorption that abuses others, is maladaptive, subjectively painful, and leaves them frustrated.

Auerbach suggests that pathological narcissism is an impairment in representational constancy. The ability to evoke images of a cohesive self and a constant object is seen as emerging in the second year of life. Although narcissistic personalities can evoke the images, this is carried out in a way that involves either a grandiose self and a depleted object, or an idealized object and a relatively empty self. The difficulty lies in making adaptive transitions between subjective and objective forms of self-awareness. In the former, the person is the center of activity, whereas in the latter, the person is one among many. These are different views of the self that create tension and a sense of division within the self. This is defended against by narcissistic fantasies that include omnipotence as subjective self-awareness and is reflected in subjective self-awareness, or merger, reflected in objective self-awareness. Normal narcissism appears as a temporary defense that passes with the integration of the two perspectives of self-reflexivity. Pathological narcissism as displayed by either a predominantly shame-prone or grandiose personality appears with increasing difficulty in self-reflexive integration. These are extreme types and there will be gradations with variable self-esteem.

These patterns have been related to the emphasis given by Kernberg and Kohut to features of narcissistic pathology. Kernberg stress grandiosity and entitlement which fits with subjective self-awareness, whereas Kohut takes note of vulnerability, inadequacy, and shame, corresponding to objective self-awareness, although both Kernberg and Kohut are aware of the presence of all these features as narcissistic pathology.

Auerbach suggests that in the anal period the child experiences a sense of separateness and vulnerability, and a limited sense of efficacy that results in a feeling of shame motivating narcissistic illusions. These can reduce the shame by self-inflation and a decreased connection to the objects, or by increasing attachment and self-effacement, as well as by variable and shifting mixtures of these positions. The grandiose position emphasizes subjective self-awareness by elevating self-esteem. In its normal forms it appears as assertiveness and self-enhancement, with grandiosity representing pathology. In comparison, objective self-awareness hides the self and idealizes the other. Normal manifestations are cooperation and modesty, with submissiveness as a pathological sign. The suggested etiology is primarily disturbances in preoedipal attachments, particularly during rapprochement, that foster both the direction of narcissistic illusions and the need to maintain them.

Fiscalini describes three major patterns of parent-child interactions that may eventuate in pathological narcissism. These are developed in the context of an optimal developmental situation in which the infant initially has an egocentric grandiosity as well as a tendency to idealize. These narcissistic characteristics then undergo transformation via appropriate parenting. This begins with relatively unconditional approval that becomes internalized and is followed by a more conditional approval that is attuned to developing capacities and needs. The desired result is a realistic basis for self-esteem, internalized autonomous standards, and empathy.

The first way that the process may go awry is with parents who continually disapprove and prematurely take away unconditional mirroring as well as opportunities for idealization. The child feels shame and has grandiose expectations of how he or she should be. There is a preoccupation with interpersonal security that results in self-centeredness that cannot be expressed directly yet interferes with interpersonal relationships. The narcissism tends to be hidden, with symptoms such as depression, withdrawal, or paranoid features being more apparent, but there is an underlying persistent need for self-approval.

In contrast, there are parents who provide exaggerated approval and prolong a child's egocentricity, creating an unusual view of the world. There is rejection of both the child's limitations and the child's need for developing realistic appraisals of the self and others. The narcissism appears in demanding, self-centered behaviors, in anxiety and anger when personal expectations are not met, and in feelings of inadequacy and shame if the person experiences realistic difficulties or failures. A variation on this pattern of spoiling the child is overprotectedness, restricting autonomy in favor of fostering parental idealization so that the child is fearful and dependent, in need of merger, with an underlying feeling of vulnerability.

Then there are parents who treat their child as special only to the extent that certain qualities of the child enhance the parents. The rest of the child is essentially ignored, with only the false self given praise and recognition. The child then feels both special yet unworthwhile, with no avenue for personal integration. The results are anger and demands for specialness because interpersonal security revolves around experiencing the self as special. However, the opportunities for that specialness are limited with the real self being unacceptable, so there are consistent needs to defend an imagined, superior self.

These types, namely the shamed child, the two types of spoiled child, and the special child, are intermingled to varying degrees. They appear as elaborations of the previously described grandiose and self-effacing narcissists of Auerbach (1993), which in turn can be related to primary narcissistic pathologies described by Kernberg and Kohut. The etiological thrust is that parents, out of their needs, create family situations where their children are forced to defend themselves in order to adapt. These defenses, or protective character styles, are distorted personal perspectives which interfere with living, particularly outside of relating to the nuclear family, and within the family result in essentially false selves. The distortion of normal narcissism is clearly a process that occurs in all disorders, but the focus here is on behavior that is particularly reflective of the self-image, such as self-absorption, grandiosity, shame, self-entitlement, and idealization, that are viewed as characteristics of pathological narcissism and in turn could be designated as indicative of a narcissistic personality disorder. In this vein, Havens (1993) has depicted pathological narcissism as the love of one's perfect image, in contrast to the acceptance of one's limitations, and Fromm (1964) compares benign narcissism with malignant narcissism that involves withdrawal to the point of conviction of one's perfection.

Bach views narcissistic pathology as a particular state of consciousness in which there is an ongoing inability to integrate subjective self-awareness and objective self-awareness. There are repetitive alterations in reflective self-awareness which are attempts to establish a sense of wholeness, self-esteem, and well-being, but which actually prevent such integration. These appear in a variety of ways. For example, there may be body-image disturbances, hypochondriacal concerns, and eating problems. Split self-representations occur, with the person who is grandiose feeling vulnerable, as well as the reverse of these feelings. There also may be a preference for self-stimulation as a substitute for object-stimulation. Language tends to be used in an autocentric fashion, with words used for manipulation, such as comforting or frightening, moving away or moving closer. There are losses of flexibility in perspective, syncretism of thought and affect, and denial of boundaries, as well as possible learning disabilities. Spontaneity is limited, decisions are difficult, and mood swings are frequent, with fears of both hyperarousal and hypoarousal. There are deficits in self-constancy, object constancy, and object relations, with oscillations between apparent self-love and object-love. All of these signs or symptoms are indicative of a fundamental difficulty, whether deficit or developmental conflict, in integrating the multiplicity of perspectives of the self.

These self-perspectives can be considered as primarily a dichotomy between subjective awareness and objective awareness that in normal development are integrated as complimentary states, but remain separated in narcissistic pathology. The balance that ought to exist becomes unbalanced. If there is an overcathexis of the self, the grandiosity predominates, along with fears of object loss and the loss of reality to the point that the world has only one person, the subject. In contrast, if the object world is overcathected, there is an increasing loss of self-esteem and fears of the loss of the self until the self has been absorbed by the world and is gone. These variations are in accord with the grandiose mirroring transference and the idealizing transference suggested by Kohut, as well as the subphase shifts from fascination with personal functioning to the need for emotional replenishment described by Mahler during rapprochement, and are in accord with the findings of all the authors discussed in this section who note both grandiosity and vulnerability in the self-absorption of narcissists. Whether apparently moving away from or toward others, the person's concern is self-protection. The personal perspective is continually fragmented so that the integration of the self has to be an ongoing, unfulfilled task.

Bach suggests that pathological narcissism is largely a result of disturbances in the preoedipal mother-child relationships. These may be an absence of dialogue, a maternal monologue, or a pseudodialogue, all of which results in the lack of empathic responsiveness and a deficiency in mother-child homeostasis. This deficiency may also occur whenever either parent should provide the function of tension regulation in interaction with the child. Two identifications appear to be particularly significant. One is an identification with the symbiotic mother which would support subjective awareness and the capacity for being with others. The other is an identification with the separating mother which would support objective awareness and the capacity for autonomy. Deficits in these identifications and inabilities in integrating subjective and objective self-awareness arise from faulty parent-child interactions. The result is either an excessive emphasis on one perspective, or excessive vacillation. The personal perspective is distorted so that the self, objects, and relationships, as well as the activities of living, are all out of focus in some fashion, the narcissistic state of consciousness that we consider to be pathological narcissism.

Conclusions

The self is considered to be the total person with different manifestations present from birth, so that there is always some self-experience in process. This experience has a perspective, a form of motivational organization designed to further personal development that is designated as narcissism. The development of narcissism is a maturational process which can be seen as a component of major developmental stage theories, such as psychosexual stages, relational stages, and senses of the self. It is continuous over the life span, and particularly influenced by the presence of significant others, and by the culture.

Bach (1985) has noted that each culture develops a definition for its members of an acceptable relationship between the external world and subjective experience. Narcissism is reflected in reactions to that cultural, societal definition, as well as to the more personal definition offered by parents to their children. Butler (1990) describes psychic life as intentional in its relatedness to the world, yet this is generally a difficult process with movement toward and away from connectedness based on narcissistic shifts.

Pathological narcissism appears when the personal perspective becomes distorted and maladaptive. Although the major theories of narcissism disagree in some of their specific emphases, there is agreement as to the major characteristics of pathological self-interest appearing primarily in either grandiose or self-effacing patterns of behavior. There is also agreement that faulty parenting seems to be the primary etiological factor, so the next section of the book will consider in detail the relationship between narcissism and the family environment.

III
Fathers and Narcissism

This chapter explores the role of narcissism in the development of the father as well as the use of narcissism in the fathering process. In order to do that it is first necessary to examine the psychology of masculinity because the role of father is embedded within the concept of masculinity. Masculinity is a combination of *gender*, which is biologically determined, *gender identity*, which refers to a person's awareness of being male or female, and *gender role identity*, which is the adherence to socially constructed norms for acting as a male or female. Thus, a boy is biologically and anatomically male, and in that sense is masculine. He also develops an awareness of his body that supports the identification as a male. In addition, and subject to considerable variation, he also learns how males are expected to behave and, again to varying degrees, conforms to the social norms of masculinity. Although the origin of fathering is biologically rooted in the use of sperm, fathering tends to be a male normative expectation with most of the fathering process an enactment of the socially and psychologically constructed masculine role. Narcissism is a significant part of both the role construction and its activation.

Masculinity

Psychoanalytic developmental psychology, particularly in its earlier forms, has often been considered as phallocentric with a positive bias toward males and their attributes. However, neither men nor women received the distinctive attention that would facilitate greater understanding of gender differences and similarities. Women were the first to redress this limitation, and recently psychologies of men have also been developed (Fogel, Lane, & Liebert, 1986; Levant & Pollack, 1995) which provide considerable information about masculinity and the contemporary role of the father.

It has become apparent that there are *masculinities*, rather than a single masculine standard, and that standards vary based on social class, race, ethnicity, sexual orientation, history, and stages of life (Kimmel & Messner, 1992). For example, Lazur and Majors (1995) describe the "cool pose" of African-American males, the machismo code of Latino men, the traditions of American-Indian males, and the privacy of Asian-American men, although noting individual differences within these groups which are reflections of personal modifications. Lazur and Majors refer to each man's "conversation with the culture" (1995, p.40) through which men uniquely operationalize gender role norms. This is another way of describing the role of narcissism in the manifestation of masculinity.

At the same time, there tends to be a dominant view which at the moment represents both a traditional ideology as well as reactions to it. The traditional masculinity is represented by a constellation that includes achievement, strength, risk taking, violence and avoidance of anything that might be considered feminine (Levant, 1996). Additional specific traits are difficulties in experiencing emotional empathy, in identifying and experiencing emotional states, in emotional intimacy, and in being equal partners with wives in home maintenance and child-rearing, as well as tendencies to turn anger into rage and violence, and to experience sexuality as distinct from relating (Brooks & Silverstein, 1995). Lest the tradition seem totally negative, Levant (1995) notes that it does have the positive components of protectiveness, loyalty, problem solving, and assertiveness.

The traditional masculinity appears to remain strong among working-class and lower class men, with some shifts for middle- and upper-middle class men. The latter groups tend not to adhere to the norms of avoiding femininity, restricting emotionality, nonrelational sexuality, and success at all costs, but they continue to endorse aggression and self-reliance (Levant, 1995). Pleck (1995) notes that although there are many masculine ideologies, it is also apparent that despite the diversity the culture still frequently supports emotional control, achievement, homophobia, and antifemininity.

In terms of reactions to the masculine tradition, the ideology of the "tough male" causes considerable conflict for everybody concerned, women, children, and men themselves. The feminist perspective that has developed has altered phallocentric theories of development (Chodorow, 1989; Jordan, Kaplan, Miller, Stiver, & Surrey, 1991), and the reappraisal of sexual identities alters traditional views of masculinity

(Domenici & Lesser, 1995). The increase in families where both parents work has changed the division of labor in and out of the household, and changed the traditional roles of father as provider and mother as caretaker. Pleck (1981, 1995) has described a gender-role strain for males as they struggle to fulfill gender role norms. The result he suggests is a marked amount of discrepancy, trauma, and dysfunction that supports the need for a redefinition of masculinity and questions the idea that men have an intrinsic psychological male identity. In such questioning, core gender identity (being male or female) is differentiated from gender role identity. The later is depicted as a more complex construct that involves each person making a decision as to what it means to be a man or a woman. These decisions are shaped by biological, social, and psychological factors. For example, Archer (1996) reviews the explanatory evidence for sex differences in social behavior from the perspective of social role theory and sexual selection theory. He concludes that the most useful approach is a coevolutionary one that takes into account gene-culture interactions. This is consistent with the biosocial theory of personality development (Harris, 1995). Within this approach the male conflict is illustrated in the emphasis on toughness and self-reliance as a component of both gendered social learning and evolutionary fitness that at the same time are displayed within a context offering many choices including entirely different behaviors that are nonetheless open to men. Thus the personal perspective is a significant interactive influence in determining gender role identity.

Contemporary psychoanalytic theory tends to give less emphasis to biological or evolutionary etiologies for gender differentiation and instead stress the role of identification. Kernberg (1976) described identification as part of a developmental line of internalized object relations. Introjection was the first step in the line followed by identification. In the latter an emphasis was given to the role of the introjected object, so that identification was equated with role internalization, and was followed by ego identity, namely organizing introjections and identifications. Incorporation, symbiosis, and merger appear as aspects of identification as well, and Benjamin (1991) points out that identification is both an internal process and a relationship.

The complexity of the gender role identification was disguised in the early psychoanalytic formulations which stressed sexual preference as the determiner of a corresponding role as a man or a woman. Anatomy indicated whether a person was a man or not and in turn the presence of a penis indicated that person would want a woman as a sexual object and would identify, via the father, with maleness and act like a man. Society was allowed to fill in the characteristics of maleness which in turn were viewed as though they automatically came with the core gender identity as biological givens.

This approach narrowed the options in the male role. Thus, Kernberg (1986) notes that homosexuality would appear as a limitation in the resolution of an oedipal situation in that the boy is expected to identify with the sexual and paternal functions of the father. However, as the concept of adaptation developed, identifications with both parents were apparent as well as sexual interests in both parents. The resolution of the oedipal situation required the boy to make a change in his early identification with the mother, and the importance of identification from infancy began to be emphasized. Prior to this two apparently contradictory features of male development had been noted, namely a constitutionally derived bisexuality and a developmental process that emphasized heterosexuality (equated with masculinity) as an obvious consequence of the anatomical differences between boys and girls. The developmental pathway for bisexuality was given limited elaboration. Its contents included wishes to be a woman in sexual relations and to bear children, but these wishes were viewed as making the boy anxious about losing his masculine identity. So the ultimate result was the limiting of the presence of a feminine identity and an emphasis on the dichotomy of the gender roles, particularly in regard to sexual preference. The reappearance of feminine identifications in males during later developmental phases was in turn viewed as regressive. This anatomical shaping of masculine identity is in sharp contrast to a more contemporary view. For example, Isay (1986) has suggested that homosexual patterns in men are a result of constitutional and developmental factors that occur early in life and that such patterns do not have to be a result of compromise formations.

An intriguing feature of bisexuality is its potential for multiple identifications. Fast (1984) conceptualizes the boy's development as involving an early identification with his mother, but in a context of masculinity so that the boy has an early nominal gender identification as a male that coexists with his identification with his mother. Thus there is an assumption of both masculine and feminine traits that at the time are not distinguished as such. The earliest experience of gender is considered relatively undifferentiated, and in that sense pansexual. The boy has an inaccurate, overextended view of his identity that could be termed omnipotent in the sense of having it both ways. The narcissism of the boy extends to whatever is knowable to him. It is limited by his lack of knowledge and the immaturities of development, yet it is unlimited by these very same features because he has yet to learn some significant limits.

Gender differentiation is viewed as starting when there is a recognition of limits that are imposed by anatomical differences so the age of this will vary. Narcissism plays a role here, along with maturational capacities, because it is not only noticing differences, but the differences have to develop a meaning. The significance of the differences, once recognized, is viewed as generating a feeling of loss in the boy's own capacities so that there is a change in his self-representation. Masculinity becomes redefined in relation to the members of the other gender who have different attributes and capacities. Narcissism can play a major role in deciding whether the boy's emphasis will be on his perceived loss or the losses of the other gender. Dahl (1988) notes that gender identity is a product of complex configurations of fantasy, with gender as a process that favors one attribute over another, not automatically focusing on what may be lost or gained in differentiation.

In Fast's conceptualization, biological factors are thought to be of limited importance per se, the emphasis being on the social meaning of the anatomical differences. The boy does not have to disidentify with his mother, as Greenson (1968) had suggested and as been described in the psychic wounding theories of male development (Bergman, 1995), or even disavow identifications with her. Instead, he differentiates his self-representations and organizes his experiences accordingly and subjectively. For example, identifying with the mother's nurturing role can certainly be included in the concept of masculinity. A feminine stage in boys is seen as an appropriate part of gender differentiation and means that other-sex characteristics are valued and their loss viewed as a narcissistic injury. However, the injury is healed and the feelings of loss replaced through a complementary notion of masculinity and a positive acceptance of gender-appropriate roles.

In the Oedipal situation the parents appear as models of masculinity and femininity, as well as reference points for testing out what it means to be male or female. The initial notions of being male or female may have been dichotomies, with defensive repudiations, but the notions are modified with certain integrations of identifications. Thus envy and anxiety are included in the developmental process of gender role identity, but are not crucial determinants. In the Oedipal period the boy tests numerous previously determined notions of masculinity and femininity that have been based on earlier identifications with both parents. The boy separates the maternal identifications that are not compatible with his emerging sense of masculinity that is greatly influenced by his father as a model. The relationships between mother and father, as well as between the parents and their son, also serve as possible models for male-female relationships.

The gender differentiation approach offers the possibility that boys utilize their increasing developmental awareness to develop characteristics that are apparently male. These characteristics include cross-sex as well as same-sex attributes. The success of this process is seen as primarily dependent on parenting that fosters a type of differentiation that provides for an integration of experienced characteristics of men and women in a complementary way that at the same time supports separate gender role identities as male or female.

Identity development is perceived as originating in primary narcissism, which is described as a type of experience which occurs interactively with the environment but is without differentiation in regard to experiencing and what is experienced. Thus narcissism is an experiential mode in which personal experience is equated with reality, involving illusions of omnipotence and primary creativity. There is a gradual differentiation of the self which at about two years of age includes the capacities for symbolic thought and recognition of a world independent of the self. The differentiations that occur include omnipotence into intention and causality, creativity into thought and what is thought about, self-other unity into self and other, and gender undifferentiation into a sex-specific self. The self is increasingly experienced as the center of individual intention and thought interacting with an independent external reality with others who are sex-specific and separate from the self. A bimodal identity is proposed with event-centered and category-centered experiences of identity that correspond to the concepts of the self as the center of experience as well as one among many. These modes of experience appear equivalent to the self-perspectives of subjective awareness and objective awareness that were previously noted as having been proposed by Bach (1985) and Auerbach (1993) as key components in the development of narcissism.

Thus infants are viewed as living within their immediate experience and perceiving all existence to be a function of the infant's experience, namely an early personal perspective that in the differentiation approach is termed infantile narcissism. Although this theory takes note of the interactive nature of infantile experience, it limits the subjective differentiation of self and other so that at first there is no sense of self or self-representation, or identification, or object representation, yet there are discrete experiences of the self interacting with the environment. The theory tries to integrate the primitive nature of thought and affect with the growth of the self without providing for a sense of self from birth, and this conception appears overly restrictive because the phrase "an experience of self" (Fast, 1984, p.115) implies some self-awareness. Also, narcissism is equated with a two year period in which differentiation develops to a point of objectification and a transition is suggested to a "post-narcissistic identity organization" (p.118) with symbolic thought, increased integration of the self and objects, and a subjective world that includes realities that are independent of the self. The categorization of narcissism as omnipotence and primary creativity that are essentially to be grown out of limits narcissism, and the terms themselves are restricted in their application to infants. Thus, a narrow view of narcissism appears in regard to the establishment of identity, which actually could be avoided by emphasizing the subjectivity of narcissism and the growth of self-reflectivity.

Also, the gender differentiation model is limited in offering motivational power for identifications. It keeps the constructs of castration anxiety and penis envy as lesser events and stresses both the reality principle of accepting the possibilities that become apparent in gender representation as well as following the patterns of one's parents, but it is not clear why those motives would be so compelling. The Oedipal situation is also resolved along conventional lines, leaving no room for other solutions as homosexuality or bisexuality as successful adaptations. Then, although a complementary gender role identity is emphasized, the ingredients of masculinity and femininity are not detailed, nor is it clear what would motivate the complementarity as opposed to the power imbalances that have customarily appeared in gender roles.

Benjamin (1995b) suggests that rather than giving up the characteristics of the other, they are retained as narcissistic potentials in one's fantasy. This facilitates living with the contradictions that continually disrupt a gendered self-representation. She asserts that it is more adaptive to view gender as transitional. Brooks and Silverstein (1995) view the differentiation model as failing to distinguish between the socialized characteristics and the biological features of gender role identity. They also express reservations about depicting gender roles in a way that espouses complementarity yet endorses considerable dichotomy, and they dispute the need for nuclear family structures to develop masculinity in boys or femininity in girls.

Pollack (1995) suggests that boys are required to separate from their mothers and give up their identification with mothers. This is experienced as a premature disruption of the holding environment, and it is made especially difficult because fathers often do not supply an adequate nurturing alternative. This causes men to attempt to create a sense of independence as a defense against reexperiencing the betrayal of dependency. Gender role socialization in schools, homes, and at work, reinforce the defensive stereotype. Bergman (1995) asserts that everything in the culture forces a boy to disconnect from a mutually empathic relationship with his mother. A relational paradox occurs in which boys disconnect to preserve themselves. Levant (1995) describes emotional socialization of boys as an "ordeal" in which mothers, fathers, and peer groups suppress and channel male emotions. The result is that men have difficulty both identifying and describing their feelings. They have *action empathy*, in that they can understand another's view in terms of what the other person will do, but lack *emotional empathy* which is an understanding of how another person feels. Anger and aggression are excessively developed and tender feelings are suppressed and channeled into sexuality.

A divisive separation from the mother during separation-individuation is seen as a common developmental trauma for boys, as is a difficult identification with fathers who are either emotionally absent or overly demanding in wanting conformity to male stereotypes. Essentially the boy is wounded before the age of three by the loss of an identification with the mother. The result is a conflictual gender role identity. The developmental trauma theory is similar to the differentiation theory in its emphasis on a core gender role identity that is destined to be restrictive, although differentiation theory does not involve disidentification from the mother. Identification is more likely a variable process for each individual, and the identification of a child with a gender role figure is tempered from the start by the expectations of the object of identification and the reciprocal reactions of the child. Thus boys and girls are likely to have different identifications with their mothers, and to process these identifications in varying ways over time. Furthermore, there is evidence that the absence of traditional parenting does not necessarily alter the development of rather conventional gender role identities in children. Two examples are children raised by lesbian partners (Patterson, 1992) and children raised in families where the fathers were primary caretakers (Pruett, 1983; Pruett & Litzenberger, 1992).

Various "signposts" pointing toward masculinity have been suggested that represent combinations of anatomy, identifications, and parental and societal attitudes along with a self-perspective. For example, Tyson (1982/1994) describes core gender identity as developing from a mixture of sex assignment at birth, biological and instinctual forces, parental behavior and early object relations, developing ego functions, and body image. The latter includes the boy discovering his penis and integrating it into the body image, which is facilitated by a relationship with the mother and the father which establishes genital awareness, defines body boundaries, and engenders castration anxiety. The father has been viewed primarily as supporting the mother but offering a nonsymbiotic relationship that facilitates separation from the mother, as well as serving the boy with an object for identification based on genital similarity. An increasing assumption of a male gender role means using the father as an ego-ideal, but the father's behavior is often a source of confusion, due to either absence or a relatively uninvolved or limited, even if controlling, role in the home. Thus, Tyson states, "the optimal situation for promoting the boy's identification with the male gender role occurs when the father is warm, affectionate, and supportive, yet is assertive, active, and constantly involved in family functioning" (1982/1984, p.183).

However, as Levant and Pollack (1995) have noted, fathers such as this have been in short supply, so the heavy reliance on identifying with the father in order to form a stable sense of masculinity is fraught with confusion. Actually, the mother as an original source of power still has a lot of appeal to the boy. The mother's attitudes toward masculinity are also very important, and are reflected in her relationship with her husband and her children. Encouragement by both parents is seen as necessary for boys to see the narcissistic value in assuming a male gender role.

Kestenberg, Marcus, Sossin, and Stevenson (1982/1994) have described masculinity and femininity as based on bisexual, biologically anchored patterns that are influenced by cultural trends, and thus adaptive. Boys are depicted as seeing their fathers as more active and aggressive thereby fostering differentiation. However, through the sensations and experiences of inner-genitality there is an identification with the mother which is balanced by an outer-genitality that includes identification with the apparent self-sufficiency of the father. There is also competition with the father, and sensuality that can come about through identification with both parents, as well as sublimations found in work. Thus the perspective is broadened to account more for a familial identification, although with considerable role demarcation based primarily on identification with the father and the mother.

Lansky (1989) expands masculine identification to include the parental imago, which functions as a representative model of both parents. The father is the socially expected model for the boy who actually internalizes the entire family. The masculine self of the boy is customarily defined by the father in relation to the mother and to any other family members, particularly siblings. Images of one parent always contain information about the other parent and about their relationship, with memory concealing as well as revealing. Thus the identifications that take place go beyond dyadic interactions and actual transitions. Integrating object relations, family group relations, and systems, Muir (1989) suggests that there is an encoding of relational systems as part of identity formation. Thus, not only will dyadic relationships be internalized, father as the male role model for example, but also the relational system of the entire family.

Bem (1993) contends that gender identity has been depicted as a product of biological essentialism, gender polarization, and androcentrism. Essentialism makes masculinity and femininity the natural consequences of biology, and gender polarization makes male-female distinctions an organizing principle for society. Finally, androcentrism creates the perspective that male experience is the norm. A biohistorical view illustrates that there has been a division of labor and power based on gender that had made men primarily providers and protectors with women as nurturers. Although this society provides a variety of possibilities for gender role identities, it narrows the acceptability of options, so that the usual result is what Bem describes as a "gendered personality," namely "a particular collection of masculine or feminine traits and a way of construing reality that itself constructs those traits" (1993,p.152).

Traditionally agenetic (individual concern) and instrumental (problem solving) traits have been considered masculine, although complementary to being communal and expressive, which were depicted as feminine. The masculine self (as well as the feminine self) are combined products of culture construction, social practices, and self-development. There is an assumed and socially enforced "natural" connection between biology and gender role identity that makes it difficult for anyone who does not conform. Thus, the general task of men is to learn the culturally acceptable definition of masculinity and to try to act accordingly. The role of enculturation is highlighted, and exposes the burden and limitations of traditional masculinity. What once may have been adaptive became entrenched regardless of its restrictions, and as questions are raised to its continuing value, the boy and his parents are faced with considerably more complexity as to what it means to be male beyond biological characteristics. David and Brannon in 1976 described normative masculinity as including emotional stoicism, aggression, physical virility, competition, achievement, and avoidance of the feminine. As Pleck (1995) notes, men have had trouble with such a role for quite a while, and it is not about to get easier, as the traditional clashes within itself, as well as with evidence that weakens or dissolves biological ties (Bem, 1993) as well as the many possibilities in gender equality. The case for the reconstruction of masculinity, and an anything-but-normative conception, is clearly being advocated (Levant, 1995).

Brooks and Silverstein (1995) propose an interactive systems model that includes social, cultural, psychological and political influences on the development of masculinity. They argue that although mothers and sons break their early attachment, while fathers and sons are emotionally separated from each other, the conflict in a boy's sense of masculinity is due to cultural restriction rather than disrupted identification. The disturbances in male behavior, such as excessive violence, are considered symptoms of role stress. This stress appears due to ecological and cultural expectations for men to take risks, compete, and be emotionally detached, essentially giving up the self and open to the abuse of power. The appeal of such a personal perspective appears to be societal approval, but the emphasis on systems also seems to ignore the diversity of personal motivations that are becoming more apparent in non-traditional male behaviors and attitudes.

Integrating Masculinity

The formation of identity includes a subjective congruence between anatomy and behavior. The anatomy of the male provides primary and secondary sexual characteristics as well as weight and height distributions and assorted physiological characteristics that are potentials for maleness. There are traditional and nontraditional ways to use these characteristics. History has played a role in deciding what was adaptive, such as the male using physical strength and displaying or containing certain emotions in stress situations. Although males are certainly not equal in either their physical potentials or the actualization of them, over time they as a group have been powerful enough to establish androcentric societies in most of the world and essentially live by the rules of force. Given that war and violence are always going on somewhere, there is considerable support for the desire for control and the presence of conflict between people, as well as the desire for sharing and harmonious living. Although Freud's duality of human nature has had numerous specific criticisms, its ongoing presence continues to be detected in major areas of life such as poverty (Herron & Javier, 1996) and ethnic tension (Herron, 1995; Javier, Herron, & Yanos, 1995). Thus males are born into a duality of personality characteristics, essentially the constructive and the destructive, with narcissism as the representation of their personal balancing act.

The existence of this duality from birth is basically argued on interpretive grounds. For example, the cry of the hungry infant can be viewed as a sign of affection or a bonding desire, yet it may well be both. It is certainly a demand of some sort, and it is destructive of whatever else the person who meets the demand was doing when the demand arrived, just as it is constructive in its appeal to another who wishes to make the connection. Furthermore, as Winnicott (1965) has deftly pointed out, infants sometimes want to be left alone, and so do adults. Thus we are all selective in our need for contact, and we are living with needs to love and destroy, because these represent our modes of taking care of ourselves, our paths to growth and self-development.

Given the birth of the male child into a currently androcentric society, the environment will be most conducive for the boy to try to follow the model of traditional masculinity. However, this does not mean that the boy will automatically fall into line, or that he should. His personal perspective will be based on what feels best for him. As Pleck (1981) has pointed out, the traditional male role is often attempted but infrequently followed completely. Anatomy and physiology may not be that cooperative as far as strength goes, and the repression of affect involved may be too taxing. In regard to identification, the assumption of a male role involves a variety of partial identifications derived from parents and other significant figures who appear to the child to have desirable features. It is, however, not the literal mother or father that is identified with, although incorporation and introjection may at first feel concrete to the child as though he is that person (or at least a body part of that person), but it is ultimately the symbolism of the parent and the significant others that represent the identification. Thus the boy child can take on whatever qualities he desires, such as nurturance, but with the differentiation that he is a nurturant *male*. As Fast (1984) notes, then certain abilities belong only to males, and other abilities are missing, or given up if the child thought he had them in the first place. The degree to which the male child experiences himself as being like the mother may include merger experiences, as well as obliterating the mother to incorporate her functions, but the ongoing process will produce essentially many partial identifications. The process of differentiation will be operative from birth, and the boy will continually be told from birth that he differs from the mother in gendered terms. His named identity will be "boy," but her designation will be "woman." At the same time, parents and families vary in the degree to which they emphasize gendered identifications, so qualities possessed by either or both parents can become part of a male identification. In essence, the boy will test out what works for him, and try to put that into effect. Certainly, parents and others will usually try to move the boy in a direction they consider to be masculine, but that does not mean he has to follow their leads. He does have to understand what boys and men usually do in this society, and be aware that there are consequences to doing the unusual. Sexual orientation is probably the most dramatic example of this, because this society discriminates against homosexuals. Physical strength is a useful attribute, but men do not all have it to the same degree. It is not essential to being a man, nor is much else, although the ways of "acting like a man" are conventionally known. Some are appealing and useful, some are appealing and harmful, and some are unappealing. In that mix, some are attainable by many, some are attainable only by a few.

In essence, being a male is one part of a personal identity, one part of who one is. Its form, beyond the anatomy, is environmentally shaped, but has a reciprocity to it as well because of the individual feelings involved. A male can feel whatever way he wants about having a penis, but the immutable is that he has one, and that gives him a certain potential for pleasure, behavior, and fantasy. The use of the penis is much more of a personal style, particularly to the degree to which anatomy is allowed to represent personality. In the process of identification, the body parts, their function and their symbolism all have played a part, and in an androcentric culture the erect phallus has stood for power. However, the essence of that power is really the performance of a sexual function. This is pleasurable, useful, and something to be missed if it were not operative, but it is not a guarantee of any other power or strength. As a result, boys learn that having a penis does not automatically make their fathers a particular way, nor will it so powerfully influence them. At the same time, it is good to have and definitely part of their identity.

The identification with masculinity is fostered in terms of the degree of gender differentiation that is appropriate to the society. It is not necessary that the boy be separated from the mother in the sense of severing a close relationship with her, but it is necessary that the relationship have boundaries, such as the lack of incest and the understanding that the boy will not be a biological mother. The initial differentiation between the infant and the mother is limited so that there can be the coexistence of ideas of being and not being the mother, as well as being and not being other significant figures. However, as differentiation increases a sense of distinctiveness accompanies a sense of connection. Connections with the mother and father are reshaped around both anatomy and function. The boy is taught and learns that he is supposed to be more similar to his father than to his mother. However, the similarity is primarily biological, although customarily the parents and society have added specific qualities to the anatomical likeness and created a constellation of traits and behaviors that are deemed masculine. The specifics of this masculinity have been developed over time in response to various environmentally adaptive needs, but they are open to change.

The shaping of identity in regard to being male does mean that the infant boy loses the possibility of being a woman and a mother. Although being mother is an anatomical illogicality that is contradicted by his designation from birth as a boy, it is a partial loss of identity that was based on a powerful connection at an early age. The value in shifting to the father is not automatically apparent. The parents play a key role in forming this transition by developing relationships with the infant that take into account gender identity. Ideally close relationships with both parents will be fostered from birth so that the infant can feel strongly connected to the qualities of each parent. The parents have the opportunity to instill pride in the child's gender identity, and therefore support its incorporation by including the obvious aspects, such as having a penis as well as having a name, in their dialogue with the child. The parents also have the opportunity to indicate the paths taken in the culture, as well as other options, and the problems inherent in sexism, as well as the possibilities of interest in sexual differentiation.

Neubauer (1986) makes the point that there are of course very significant primary parental objects, but there are also multiple object relationships. Anatomy, family, drives, society, and relationships are all intermingled as potential gender role identity influences, but it is the personal perspective, the narcissism of the self that ultimately makes an integration, follows a primary direction, and proposes a definition, a "this is me, I am a man." The content of that definition is our next concern.

The Content of Masculinity

The ingredients of the male gender role, namely the set of rules by which men were to operate, were always subjectively experienced and defined. However, the idea that nature played a more significant role than nurture tended to dominate descriptions and prescriptions for males. The range of approved narcissistic possibilities was relatively limited. Sexual preference was mandated heterosexual, and role behaviors such as aggression, strength, and success were considered normative expectations. Deviations, such as homosexuality, passivity, weakness, and a lack of ambition were met with derision and social sanction. Many if not most men failed in one or more of the main goals of their gender role, but they were expected to keep trying.

This content of masculinity was learned both from anatomical possibilities, such as the function of a penis or the use of physical skills, and from caretakers and the larger society. Thus a personal perspective that differed from what was expected was not reinforced, or it was undermined, or denied by parents as well as by the developing individual, creating a conflict for anyone outside the norm, which ended up including most men to varying degrees. The narcissistic ego ideal for many men was the functional ideal of society for men. However, as Erikson (1968) suggested, cultural processes, and individual ones have a type of interpenetrability and mutual influence, so that in time there are few if any fixed functions. Gender provides certain boundaries as well as certain possibilities, but Fast (1984) has emphasized the complementary nature of gender. The subjectivity of gender roles is becoming more apparent, so that the narcissism of gender role identity has more possibilities. There are more and more different ways to identify the self as male, that although including anatomy, do not have anatomical destinies.

The idea of identifying with the father has always been a major conception in explaining the acquisition of a masculine identity, but fathers are usually less present as caretakers than mothers. As a result, it is often the role of the mother to make the abstract father, and in turn the absent male, a desired object for boys. Single parent families are usually headed by mothers, and intact families that rely heavily on child care usually get it from females, so a major directive force for boys is a woman's view of masculinity. The father of course can fill in specifics and be more of a presence than he has been in the past, but this involves an expansion of the father's narcissism to provide active identification from birth, which is usually not the case (Lamb, 1977; Neubauer, 1986). What appears to happen is that there are limited, partial, and oscillating identifications with both parental figures, as well as with other caretakers, peers, and other figures of interest which strike responsive chords within the individual and which ultimately coalesce into an identity that includes a gender role. Because of their experience with society, the major caretakers generally try to develop the child according to an adaptive role, to make a fit between anatomy and the cultural expectation that the caretakers are familiar with. This need not be an inflexible fit however, nor is it guaranteed to be one of the child's liking. It is primarily a role selected by the parents for reasons of their own, and it is undergoing considerable reconceptualization.

Thus prevailing postmodernism offers less certainty but more possibility. One can become a person who also is a man, rather than a man who is also a person. This does not mean that there are no values in gender differentiation, but it does negate the traditional male superiority, privilege, and normativeness. The differences that are of value, such as complementarity and enjoyment of particular functions, are there to be developed, while the differences of bias are ripe for elimination, as the feminist movement has made particularly clear.

Criticism of past (and often still prevailing) versions of masculinity and opportunities for enlightenment and change pose threats and confusion to an established order that many people still find attractive. How many is a difficult question to answer because research samples are not sufficiently representative of the population to say how much change is really afoot and how well it is being received. Political correctness and "real selves" are not necessarily in concordance, but it is clear that the male gender role has undergone some changes. A major alteration has been the great increase in families where both parents work. This changes the division of labor, particularly traditional roles of male provider and female caretaker, and in turn the role models. However, (Brooks & Gilbert, 1995), this has often resulted in the mother doing double duty, as well as both partners having mixed feelings about shifting roles, but the boy would not automatically identify with the provider role as a masculine prerogative or necessity.

The narcissism of the child is drawn to the major motivations that have been suggested in the evolution of psychoanalytic theory, as pleasure, safety, love, contact, and cohesion. There is also a growing awareness of the need for action to derive sought after reactions, and an awareness of "boyness" that is akin to "relatedness" in the integration of an identity. Thus the boy-man is partially identified by his body, and in that sense can most easily identify with his father and other males. His feelings about the identification will vary in terms of the degree of acceptance and pleasure in having a male anatomy and the use he makes of the anatomy, but unless he changes the anatomy, which happens in only a small number of instances, he will try to make the most adaptive use of it. The rest of the male identity, and that is a very substantial portion, provides more options for expression, although there are social superego-type boundaries there that get stretched or broken only at some affective cost. Power-sharing, for example, is behavior that some males will resist because they see no personal advantage to it. At the same time, the idea that because one is male means one must be powerful can be a burden that some males would prefer not to have.

The presence of "gender strain" in regard to fulfilling the male gender role highlights the narcissistic conflict. Narcissism sends the message of getting your needs met, and then needs often become conflictual. Healthy male narcissism deletes the small incremental gains of momentary satisfaction in favor of a broader personal perspective of personal integrity and respect. The warrior is the caretaker. However, the male world is by custom a violent, aggressive place, and it takes considerable courage and wisdom to feel comfortable as a man. There are of course many pathways to more loving societies, but the course of history argues against any of them gaining such ascendance that males will any time soon be relieved of either the burden or the enjoyment of being the warrior. However, it is also unlikely that male caretaking will decrease, or that males will be encouraged to be less sensitive or less connected to others than they already are. Male narcissism needs to be opened up to more behavioral and affective possibilities.

The male can best be aided in the development of his identity by understanding that there are in a sense no roles that have to be assumed to be a male, as well as that there are adaptive consequences in choosing how to display a masculine role. In addition, it is clear that characteristics such as empathy and intersubjectivity are valuable narcissistic attributes for men, particularly when it comes to being a father, a role that is likely to remain prominent in present as well as future male gender role identification. Thus, in the next section we turn to the narcissism of the father, namely his subjectivity or personal perspective as demonstrated in the process of parenting.

Fathering

Being a father has just never gotten the attention in the psychoanalytic literature, or even in developmental theory in general, that has been given to being a mother. The power of a father was stressed in the Oedipal period, and note was taken of the preoedipal father as a representative of reality, and a useful "other" from the mother, particularly in fostering male identifications. The mother appeared to have the task of providing for female identification, and the father for male, although the key role played by the mother in fostering male gender role identity and the father's role in developing female gender role identity for his daughters have become more apparent.

Rotundo (1993) notes that before the 18th century there was a patriarchal system in which fathers were the primary source of leadership and moral instruction, and most of their attention was focused on the sons. Then into the early 19th century the father's role narrowed to the provider role with limited participation in family life and the responsibility for the children became primarily the mother's. Rotundo (1987) notes that fathers then tended to be detached from their sons, with more emotional involvement with their daughters. Pleck (1987) saw another change between 1946 and 1965 with the father being viewed as a model for male identification, but at the same time the father came to be seen as an often-absent figure, both physically and psychologically, who as a result contributed significantly to insecure male identities in sons. This time has been followed by a focus on the "involved father" who is a definite emotional and physical presence within the family. This has been accompanied by an interest in the preoedipal father (Ross 1982/1994) as compared to the previous images of the primarily oedipal father, and has emphasized the need to recognize and understand the father's role throughout the child's development.

What has customarily been expected of a father? Brooks and Gilbert (1995) have suggested a number of major roles that could still be considered the mainstream expectations. The first of these is being a provider, which could be currently modified to being one of the providers, although usually the major one. Thus the growing boy learns to identify with the provider role and views his significance in the family as a substantial provider, giving his wife and children what they need, often with the view of giving them more than he had himself. This attitude is most easily adopted in intact families with a good amount of cohesion, and is subject to more variations where either the parents have separated so that "provision" is an issue, or where there is antagonism between family members, and the degree of providing becomes a weapon that is used to attack each other. Thus there are many possible exceptions to the provider role. For example, for some men being a father simply means the cocreation of a child, without adding any responsibility for the child once conception takes place. Thus, making children becomes a sign of potency and virility, but there is little or no interest in the child after that. This is a view that is opposed to both legal and ethical rules, but does exist and illustrates how the narcissism of the father is involved. Essentially, it means the personal view that the man has developed in regard to what "fathering" means.

The more customary view is that a father is responsible for the care of his children until they become adults. This responsibility is usually translated into being the monetary support and has often been equated by fathers with a display of love for their families. Sometimes it is given without regard for the degree of gratitude shown by the family members, but at other times it becomes contingent on how much the children appear to love the father. A superego aspect can also be at work here, in terms of deciding what is the "right" amount of provision, namely what feels correct to the father, so that some fathers emphasize provision and even "buy love," whereas others limit it on the grounds of "the best thing for the child."

For all fathers, there is the question, what am I going to get out of being the provider? The usual forms of satisfaction are gratitude, love, respect, power, and approval. The provider role has been designated as the correct thing as well as the role that puts and keeps the father in control. As women become more significant providers the value of the role for fathers is threatened and is undergoing renegotiation. Also, as children observe family arrangements where the father is not that much of a provider, the children will also question how essential that role is to fathering. The essence of fathering is providing part of the child care, basically the amount and kind needed that is agreed upon by the entire family. This is a process that is generally worked out between the parents, with increasing input from children as they become more aware of their needs and capable of making a case for them. In non-intact families, there is usually a legislated mother, though in practice it may become the major responsibility of the parent who is willing to meet it. It is clear, however, that it is not an inherent characteristic of fathering that the father be the sole or major provider.

Related to the provider role is the one of protector. These roles are linked because economic provision is a component of protecting family and the children from various potential disasters and limitations. However, the father is also expected to physically protect, such as going to war if necessary, and using physical force. Although physical aggression is less common as an expectation from middle-class or upper-class fathers, it remains prominent in ethnic minorities and lower-class men for whom life may actually be more physically dangerous (Majors & Billson, 1992; Mirande, 1985). Also, Brooks and Silverstein (1995) have shown how violence is strongly embedded in the masculine image, so that it becomes accessible in the role of protecting father. At the same time, the aggression of protection frequently gets used as an expression of power in the abuse of children and wives.

Even when physical toughness is not emphasized, emotional toughness generally is, so that fathers can construe their roles as stoic leaders of the family whose views will be given priority. The emotional and physical toughness is often combined with disdain for the "feminine," the latter being equated with emotionality and vulnerability. Of course, as mothers have increasingly carried out provider and protector roles along with nurturing ones, it is clear that fathering can still involve the traditional roles, but it does not have to, nor does it have to be so limited that other roles are avoided or denigrated.

Fathering is customarily associated with a male gender role identity which is part of the attainment of gender consistency, and represents creativity or generativity by the male. This gender constancy begins with the categorizing of people by gender and is subsequently reinforced by an awareness of the immutable aspects of gender. Genital awareness and awareness of genital anatomical differences appear relatively early in development and are part of a general body outline as a male or female. However, for the male this at first is only associated with the knowledge that masculinity and fatherhood belong together. This knowledge does not include the functions of being a father.

Given the possibilities of over-inclusion, cross-gender preoedipal behavior, and the generally lesser availability of the father for identification, it is likely that fantasies of fathering are for many years part of a complex image of masculinity. Being a father is categorically limited to being a male, but many of the functions of fathering (and mothering) are not categorically gender-limited, which is a source of confusion for parents. Fathering as part of the expression of one's gender identity reflects a shifting relationship among psychic forces that is highly personalized, regardless of social forces, at the same time that it is interactive with external reality and social expectations. In that sense, then, it is always narcissistic, as the father configures and reconfigures the needs and demands that are internally and externally generated.

Colarusso (1990) suggests fathering is part of the separation-individuation processes, but the role of the mother, and the readiness to be a parent are seen as more prominent and accessible to the female. This absence of the father and the boy as father suggests a potential difficulty in the boy becoming a father. He usually begins to learn the role later in his development, and often learns it first through his mother rather than directly from his father or by personal identifications with his father. It would appear that boys are raised more to be men than fathers while girls may be raised more to be mothers than women. Feminist research and literature have made it clear that the gender role can be expanded for women, and in so doing, have also expanded the role for men. In essence, males can "mother" in many ways, so that their gender designation as father does not have to be so narrow, and the role of father, based on gender, can be reshaped as to both the fantasy and reality of its functions. Contemporary literature on masculinity is in accord with this view (Levant & Pollack, 1995). Brooks and Gilbert (1995) point out that men are increasingly involved in sharing parenting, so that the combination of work and fathering is becoming more of a family norm. Some of this is due to social change, but it is also a function of personal motivations. It is just as natural and possible for men to love children and want to be involved with them as it is for women (Gilbert, 1988), even though such a view of fathering has not been fostered and has been obscured by traditional stereotypes. Furthermore, the role of father does not have to be enjoyed in only customary family settings, but is quite applicable to divorced fathers as well as gay fathers. At issue here is the willingness of males and females to make narcissistic shifts that allow for diverse gender role identities.

From the father's perspective the child is a reproduction of the self, an extension of the self, and an opportunity for the self. The father has the possibility of bonding with the child and participating in the development of this bond that will continually change as the child develops. A variety of relationships are possible and probable between father and child, and these relationships can be relatively independent of the gender of the child. Benjamin (1991) has pointed out that the representation of the father in the preoedipal period is important for girls and boys. With traditional parenting, the father represents the recognition of independence more than attachment, although this could vary in different types of parenting. However, the father will usually be perceived in the rapprochement phase as a subject who can provide recognition through identification. The mother may also be perceived that way, but because the parents are seen as different from each other, they offer different recognition possibilities. Benjamin (1991) notes that the child might move toward the father out of a variety of needs, as separation, avoidance/ambivalence, and the representation of desire, but the success of the father-child relationship rests heavily on the reciprocity of the father. In this regard, fathers have usually given more to their sons, bypassing the fact that identification provides for emotional ties that are valuable to all children regardless of gender.

Benjamin (1988) offers a model that involves the establishment of a core gender identity between 12 and 18 months, with gender role identity developing as part of the separation-individuation process, which is in accord with the individuation processes described by Colarrusso (1990). Identifications with both parents as well as differentiation of roles is seen in the second and third years, with the role of the father gaining in importance. In line with Fast (1984), she describes the preoedipal phase as over inclusive, and ending with an awareness of gender limits as well as protesting against them, exemplified in penis and pregnancy envy as well as castration fears. In the oedipal phase, same-sex identification is strong at first, but later decreases with the possibility of cross-gender identifications.

This models mixes separation-individuation concepts with drive oriented ones, such as penis envy, but reinterprets the concepts. For example, the drive for the phallus can represent both heterosexual desire and homoerotic incorporation for identification on the part of the girl. Identification and object love are in turn then viewed as coexisting motives. As a result the role of the father includes the provision of identification for both genders as well as being an object of desire. The father, just like the mother, provides in the parent-child relationship many possibilities for the child to learn gender roles that are not closely bound to gender.

A consistent theme runs through all these accounts of gender development. The father is the "other" to the mother, but the specifics of being "other" vary for the child. They reflect personal choice within social and reality contexts. The boy's role as a father then will develop as a fit between what is needed in an actual parental relationship and the fantasy of being a father, and this fit customarily requires an integration that is adaptive and flexible. The good father then is represented by taking care of the child in such a way that mutual recognition of subjectivities is continually considered. In contemporary parenting, the healthy narcissism of the male as father is expressed in functions that are both traditional (protective) and not so traditional (nurturing), and are a product of the needs of the family as a system, as well as the dyadic relationship of father to child, father to mother, and child to mother.

The mutuality of the parents operates as a way to establish the specifics of fathering. Generally the father will appear as a significant figure to the child later in the developmental sequence than the mother, and the roles of each parent will be gendered in many ways. At the same time, the father can be willing to be available for the purposes of identification, recognition, complementing the mother, and being a significant "other" at all developmental stages, so that he is not locked into a gender role.

This healthy narcissism can break down in a variety of ways that are essentially a result of the father needing to be attentive to personal needs in a manner that is detrimental to the child. For example, the father may experience the child as a rival for the affection of the mother and the father then reacts by avoiding the child, or by being hostile to the child. Another possibility is that the father experiences the child as an opportunity to gain gratifications that he has missed, so that the father attempts to control the child's interests and behavior. The father intends to make the child into the person that he failed to be regardless of what the child wants. Whether the father is overly gratifying or overly frustrating, the emphasis is on the distorted needs of the father rather than the care of the child. Still another possibility involves the mother, who is often the depictor to the child of the image of the father. If the father is in conflict with her, or if they collude to distort the father's relationship with the child, then pathological narcissism will again be apparent in the fathering process. Atkins (1984) has pointed out how the mother's view is often a major portion of what the child considers as the experience of fathering.

Lansky (1992) notes some differences in mothering and fathering. Mothering is viewed in the context of a desire by the child to be cared for, whereas the child's desire for the father is more aligned with the reality principle. The typical father-functions are designed to help the child face the world, and constitute provision, protection, and guidance. The father's narcissistic equilibrium is viewed as dependent upon idealized aspirations of being the provider, and the pathology of narcissism is reflected in the shame at failures in meeting these aspirations. Fathers who are pathologically narcissistic are viewed as having unmet needs for selfobject functions, such as empathy and affective recognition, and view their needs as shameful, and as preventing the fathers from providing these functions to another person. They become connected to their wives and children in a system that emphasizes blaming, pathological preoccupation, and impulsive action, particularly violence. It could be construed then that any developmental conflicts or deficits that contribute to the skewing of the father's personal perspective in a way that avoids mutuality and intersubjectivity, represents pathological narcissism that will most likely be translated into pathological fathering.

Thus, if there are developmental arrests or distortions in drive expression, these may facilitate incestuous or sadistic fathering. The lack of appropriate ego functioning can contribute to defensive fathering. Difficulties in separation-individuation or in the establishment of security operations can eventuate in a replay between father and child. Problems arising from self-fragmentation have already been noted. Regardless of the main motivational emphasis for the father, the probability of repeating unresolved narcissistic issues with children is high.

In contrast, good fathering rests on personal perspectives that consider child care a rewarding, desired experience. The specifics of this will vary, undoubtedly including both traditional activities, as provision, and less traditional, as nurturing. The key element is to have narcissism that fosters an adaptive, complimentary way of functioning in a family system, including a system in which the customary partner is missing, or limited in some way, or unusual (same gender). This can be facilitated through favorable identifications with parental figures, social learning, and evolutionary psychology, but it is ultimately a matter of personal choice within a given context. Thus the healthy narcissism of the father is reflected in motivation and interest, flexibility and adaptiveness, and connection and recognition.

IV
Mothers and Narcissism

In this chapter, the focus is on narcissism in mothers and in the mothering process, beginning with an examination of femininity. The terms *gender*, *gender identity*, and *gender role identity* are defined in this chapter the same way as they were in Chapter III. Thus, a girl is feminine in the sense of being biologically and anatomically female, and she develops an awareness of her body that supports the identification as female. In addition, she learns how females are expected to behave and conforms to the social norms of femininity, although there are considerable variations in both the learning and the conformity. Although the origin of mothering is biologically grounded in the use of eggs, mothering tends to be a female normative expectation to an even greater degree than fathering is for males, and most of the mothering process is an enactment of a feminine role that is socially and psychologically constructed. Narcissism is a significant part of both constructing and activating the feminine role.

Femininity

In discussing female development the term "femininity" is being used as a category with the recognition that there are many "femininities," namely diversity within the category (Jordan, 1997c) as is true of masculinity. However, there does tend to be a mainstream view that represents both a traditional ideology as well as reactions to this view. One way in which femininity is described is as the opposite of masculinity, which has a similarly gross parallel picture in the common description of masculinity as that which is "not feminine." These are "you know what I mean" descriptions that leave a large amount of variable uncertainty up to the individual (the presence of personal perspectives even in stereotypes can be noted here). Despite the inaccuracies and indefiniteness, the point made is that men and women are pictured as basically different, the extension of biology into psychology in an extensive manner.

The specifics that go along with such an extension have been described by a number of authors. Lerner (1991) points out that women are considered dependent, passive, illogical, intellectually limited, weak, fragile, emotional, manipulative, and submissive. Parker (1995) mentions loving, receptive, sensitive, and narcissistic, as well as maternal, and points out the contradictions in mothering fitness that exist between the feminine characteristics of sensitivity, receptivity, and caring, and the feminine characteristics of passivity, weakness, and narcissism. Oakley (1980) lists dependence, passivity, ineptness, emotional lability, and sexual inhibition, and Brennan (1992) mentions aggression against the self, masochism, inactivity, daydreaming, narcissism, weak sense of justice, limited social sense and limited sublimation, repression, and rigidity. Also, although all women do not become mothers, and women appear to join men in experiencing marked ambivalence in the actual process of parenting, femininity and mothering appear more intertwined than masculinity and fathering. Parker refers to this phenomenon as the "elision of femininity of and maternity" with maternity as "the ultimate personality test for women" (1995, p. 157). Benjamin (1988) points out that in this unfortunate equation the mother is a desexualized person who is idealized as living to serve the needs of the child. Personal sexual feelings do not fit with this image. Furthermore, even when and if being a woman is separated from being a mother, the sexual woman tends to be a sexual object. Desire is expressed primarily through being desired. Benjamin states, "Women's sexual agency is often inhibited and her desire is often expressed by choosing subordination. But this situation is not inevitable;..." (1988, p. 90).

Eichenbaum and Orbach (1983) note the mixed feelings about women's bodies, exalted yet degraded, the dangerous nature of a female sexuality, and the tendency for many young women to dislike their bodies and be frightened of their sexuality. They see the psychological development of women as being shaped in the mother-daughter relationship, which already operates in a patriarchal culture. Thus, mothers and daughters are seen as sharing gender identities, social roles and expectations, and an inferior status that includes passivity, submission, and the repression/suppression of many desires in service of being accommodating to others.

Most of the characteristics of femininity that have been described thus far either sound unappealing or are viewed as relatively negative or limiting attributes, (other than from the viewpoint of those whose lives get facilitated by these "feminine" traits). Narcissism, for example, is depicted in pathological terms as selfishness rather than the personal perspective emphasized in this book. Another way of looking at cultural feminism has been suggested, namely as resistance to patriarchy (Irigaray, 1991), so that the positive nature of a number of feminine qualities are noted, such as emotional availability, relational adeptness, and controlled aggression. The work of Bakan (1966) can also be used in this way in that the masculine ideology of agency is compared with the female personality that emphasizes communion, namely contact with others. Chodorow (1994) also stresses the positive quality of women's interest in relationships and the formation of connections, and this view is dominant in the work of Jordan et al. (1991). The latter depict femininity as founded around a core self that is interested in others, empathizes, and is involved in an interactional model that provides for empowerment as well as accommodation.

Moving in this direction is helpful in developing a balanced perspective regarding a number of traditional feminine traits, but there also needs to be a way to account for the agency-aggression link. As Flax (1990) points out, the negative components of aggression, such as hate and rage, start to appear less than visible in this phallic/loving woman. Femininity, akin to masculinity, is individually so complex and replete with ambivalence, that Parker states, "Femininity is a cultural product, historically constructed with no fixed referent" (1995, p. 156).

Generally, with regard to female-male differences, situational contexts have been undervalued and biology has been overemphasized. Benjamin (1988) acknowledges that anatomy, biology, and genetics all play a significant role in developing the ingredients of femininity, but the psychological integration of these "facts of nature" are the products of social constructions developed by individuals. Thus, the role of the personal perspective can be viewed as a key factor in establishing femininity. Benjamin notes that Freud remarked that women are made, not born, and she adds, "femininity is a complex creation of unconscious mental life" (1988, p. 93).

Conventional femininity is usually presented in androcentric terms, moving beyond the anatomical facts of vagina, clitoris, and uterus to a social-psychological definition emphasizing an expressive, relational orientation, gender polarization, heterosexuality, and inferiority to men. Motherhood is often depicted as an essential desired ingredient, sexual desire is downplayed, social reality is approached in gendered terms so that there is an avoidance of being perceived as "masculine," and strength is in turn used selectively. For example, a woman is expected to be active in regard to bearing and rearing children, but passive in regard to being the primary economic provider. Women are also assigned both positive and negative aspects of their feminine qualities. For example, nurturance is viewed as helpful to those injured, yet limiting in terms of being assertive. As with masculinity, there is a social pressure on women to be gendered, so that men are continually striving to be "real men" (not feminine), while women are at work being "real women" (not masculine). However, the fact that this process is indeed "work" and continuous illustrates the conflict involved in such a polarized view of gender identity, particularly gender role identity.

Montrelay (1993) offers the possibility of a feminine unconscious that contains a concentric, nurturing femininity, and a phallic, aggressive femininity that are in conflict, resulting in considerable ambivalence. Kristiva (1989), focusing on the maternal role in female psychology, includes both love and hate. The theme is one of diversity in identity that allows room for the ambivalence noted by Parker (1995), who also stresses an appreciation of bisexuality as well as the disentanglement of maternity and femininity so that each can be better understood, and in particular the role of aggression can be appreciated as something other them maladaptive.

Psychoanalytic developmental theory, particularly in its more contemporary forms, de-emphasizes the role of biological or evolutionary forces in the establishment of the feminine personality. Gender identity is seen as a significant part of the self (Formanek, 1982) and Chodorow (1989) has noted that neither biology or socialization adequately account for the persistence of this feature of self-development. A basic consideration is that usually women are the primary caretakers of children, and that in turn, even if by proximity and frequency of contact, the mother-daughter relationship is of major importance to women. The mother, through her own identificatory needs, builds a bond with her daughter that emphasizes connection and fluid ego boundaries so that a key characteristic of the feminine personality is relating to others. Of course, the mother is also the major caretaker of her son, but the bond is thought to be different, with less of a need for the mother to identify and more of a need for her to foster masculine individuation.

Narcissism comes into play through internalization and organization by the daughter in relation to her mother primarily, although others such as the father are part of these social and identificatory relationships. Added to this are cultural expectations, but there is a unique aspect to the shaping of all experience that reflects narcissism, and gender identity is part of this developing personality. A primary identification is established between the daughter and the mother which lacks differentiation (Chodorow, 1989), and is oral-incorporative, facilitating attachment. This is followed by separation-individuation which in the case of the girl is complicated by a double identification on the mother's part in which she both identifies with her own mother in being a mother, and identifies with the child in re-experiencing herself as the child. Thus Chodorow suggests that from birth women identify more with daughters and slow their separation, a process usually reciprocated by the daughters. The meaning of femininity, operationalized, is made available to the girl on a routine basis through her interactions with her mother. Identification with what it means to be feminine as displayed by the mother is available on a continual basis and the dis-identifications that do occur are on a relatively partial basis, namely a degree of individuation as a person.

Both male and female infants are viewed as both identifying with the mother and viewing her as their initial sexual object, so that the girl will have to let a heterosexual identification prevail over a same-sex object choice to adhere to the customary resolution of the oedipal situation. The retention of the identificatory attachment to the mother is based on its intense satisfaction so that the mother is not given up as a primary libidinal choice because of a dissatisfaction with the mother, or blaming the mother for the girl's lack of a penis. Instead the father is gradually drawn into an already existing alliance with the mother that is now ambivalently expanded to include the father. The social-familial structure is learned and internalized so that the little girl will recreate the maternal-wife role which has to include the man-father as the primary libidinal choice, but without renouncing object-ties to mother and other women. The type of object cathexis is altered, but the intensity is considered stronger than the object-ties of boys to their same-sex parent, and that limitation in connection is viewed as frequently applicable to males in all their relationships, particularly those with women. Thus, the primary motivation for the female-male relationship is shifted away from an exclusive or even very strong reliance on sexual desire to an emphasis on sex-role learning as a function of fitting in with a social-familial structure. In addition to limiting the role of desire, and the role of aggression, this is strictly a heterosexual model.

A potential difficulty in connection lies in a subsequent struggle for individuation. In the oedipal situation, the girl cathects the father with greater force than in the preceding psychosexual stages, but still does not replace the mother. It is an erotic cathexis, but it is an addition rather than a substitution, with a distinction drawn between erotic and emotional attachments and a probability of a strong, even primary emotional attachment remaining to the mother. Chodorow (1989) suggests that the father as an erotic object is chosen more as part of the mother-daughter relationship than out of a biological desire. In essence, it is more of a relational issue than a body issue. The narcissism that is involved appears in the service of wanting to be like the mother, with a strong degree of identification that mitigates concepts such as rivalry, displacement, and ambivalence.

The differentiation of self from others is also perceived as revolving primarily around the mother. The father is significantly less an object of early symbiosis/identification because he appears more separate by virtue of being less of an early caretaker. It is the recognition of the mother's separate interests that accentuates the existence of a separate self for the girl. The mother is depicted as posing both the original threat to narcissism (intrusion via unity) and the original support of narcissism (survival through dependence). Thus, another reason to limit erotic love for the mother is to avoid a loss of desired ego boundaries, and the father can be used without that threat because his cathexis limits dependence on the mother. There appears to be a stronger need on the girl's part to be loved by the father than to love the father, resulting in an idealization of the father that permits love to appear toward him. His love for her emphasizes her distinctiveness to complement the more maternally narcissistic love from her mother. The girl tends to enter the oedipal situation later than the boy, and develops with a greater concern than the boy for both internal and external object relationships. The resolution of the oedipal triangle actually involves a retention of triadic relationships in which the relationship to men is more utilitarian than exclusive and affective relationships with the mother and other women are primary.

The reformulation of psychoanalytic theories of feminine development by Chodorow (1989) are particularly significant in charting the course of understanding contemporary theories of femininity. First, there is a focus on people being inherently social and intersubjective.

Then, there is a significant concern with mother-daughter identifications, and identifications as relationships. Then, there is a comparison of the development of males and females that exposes the limitations of an androcentric, phallocentric bias, and in so doing highlights both the struggles of men to achieve satisfactory relations as well as the relational advantages possible for women.

Chodorow (1989) held that in the context of the mother being the primary parent for all children, men and women developed different self-concepts that included different gender identities. The basic feminine self emphasizes connection, self-in-relationship, and mothering, whereas the basic masculine self focuses on separation, self-in-isolation, and makes fathering a relative after-thought that happens to come along with the need for women as libidinal outlets. The inner world of women is seen as more complex and relational than that of men, who are viewed as more defensive. Also, a rather vibrant bisexuality is seen in women relative to men, although the libidinal quality of it stresses feeling more than instinctual desire. This implies a differentiation of both libido and aggression into relational and narcissistic (autonomous) categories, although this distinction is not clearly articulated. The role of aggression appears in negative reactions to women, particularly to the mother, and to femininity, which are seen in both genders, but primarily in men, and which are considered responsible for male dominance in society, and for tension in male-female relationships. Although, the development of masculinity is seen as more difficult than femininity, the relational self of women is seen as prone to both assets, such as nurturance, and liabilities, such as dependence. Genital differences, and in turn, body-image, are not seen as essential to gender identity, but relations are, particularly the mother-child relationship. When narcissism is described, the theory wavers. Sometimes narcissism seems to be positioned in contrast to object relations, but at other times, a "relational narcissism" is more apparent. However, the emphasis on self-development, internalizations and personal alterations of relationships, can be construed as seeing femininity as a personally constructed concept, that although relationally and culturally interactive, remains basically subjective.

Revisiting Freud

Psychoanalytic theories of gender identity are customarily developed in relation to Freud's original formulations. In Freud's conceptions there is an emphasis on the meaning of anatomy that is apparently given significant recognition in the phallic phase, with anatomical distinctions relatively unrecognized prior to that time, but with a slant in the direction of a masculine unisexuality. It is a shift in libido from orality and anality to the genitals that provides an active desire for the mother, exemplified in masturbation, clitoral for the female. This concentration of libidinal genitality also involves comparison of genitals, and the girl's discovery of the absence of a penis, as well as a desire for it. The clitoris is viewed as inferior, both in term of size and gratification, and she envies the penis as well as becoming angry at her mother for having deprived her of the penis. She turns to her father in the hope of getting a penis and a penis-baby from him, and there is the oedipal situation. In its resolution the girl gives up her active pursuit of the mother as a sexual object and instead identifies with the mother as one who seeks out the male as a love object and does this through emphasizing the vagina rather than the clitoris, as well as being someone who gets back the lost object via the male's penis and the possibility of a baby.

This was never a particularly satisfactory explanation for feminine gender identity. Early challenges appeared in the works of Melanie Klein (1932) and Karen Horney (1933). Klein put more emphasis on pre-oedipal development, aggression, and object relations, but retained such concepts and drives as motivational. Reformulating Freud while remaining essentially connected to his concepts became one way to develop a new view of feminine development (Glover & Mendell, 1982; Tyson, 1994).

These revisions involve a reinterpretation of libidinal and aggressive drive components in the formation of a feminine identity. Shifts in the centrality of certain concepts, such as the importance of the discovery of sexual differences between boys and girls, tend to make these reformulations awkward when an integration is attempted with the usual way of viewing the oedipal conflict and resolution. So, for example, if girls and boys have relatively parallel paths of differentiated gender identity, the elements of the oedipal situation are also altered. A key feature in this process is the concept of identification. Glover and Mendell (1982) note that identification is a change in the self representation that includes some parts of the object representation. Thus from the origins of the formulation of representation there is a process of multiple and shifting selective identification, including ongoing dis-identification as well as re-identification. The numerous possibilities involved in the processes of identification were noted a while ago by

Jacobson (1964) when she distinguished between total identification as a union with the mother and identification with selective qualities of the love object. Bergmann (1982) takes the issue much further when she postulates identifications of different intensity with either parent as oedipal relations. This is a key because an appropriate understanding of both femininity and masculinity has to take into account possibilities of appropriate gender identities developing in a variety of ways. In the reformulations suggested thus far, heterosexuality remains as the normative path for being either masculine or feminine, which unfortunately tends to pathologize other preferences and outcomes.

These reformulations are nonetheless particularly significant in moving the understanding of feminine development into a space of its own. This is reflected in the differentiation model proposed by Fast (1984) in which marked attention is paid to the workings of identifications, but where narcissism continues to be used overtly as a counterforce to object relations. However, all of the preoedipal revisions described up to this point emphasize a personal perspective, but they do not call it narcissism.

Differentiation

The differentiation hypothesis is that gender identity is one of a number of developmental potentials that originate in undifferentiated states. In this case, at first the girl's sense of herself is not limited by her gender, but then there is a recognition of a sex difference, with the penis as a focus for a sense of loss. However, the loss is one of unlimited possibilities, and now experience is reorganized in gendered terms. Female genitality is integrated as part of her body image and femininity, whereas male genitality is ascribed to boys and considered reciprocal. A wish for a baby expresses both identification with the mother, and an expected relationship with the father now that the parents are also reconceptualized along the lines of their gender identity. The process of gender differentiation is depicted by Fast (1984) as overcoming narcissism, which is equated with a sense of omnipotence and overinclusion. From birth there have been indications of female identity, including genital sensations and social influences. At the end of her first year, differential relationships are established to the father and mother, and femininity and masculinity are attributed to the self and others by about age two. Fast (1984) does not dispute the sense of loss at observing that a boy has a penis and the girl does not, but views penis envy and a desire for a penis as representing a desire for having everything rather than having maleness. The male is seen now as also limited, because he is different, and it is the difference itself that changes the object world into gendered terms.

The restructuring of the self and object worlds that occurs involves an increase in genital interests that has a foundation of both social and bodily experience. Emphasis is given to a recognition and understanding of the limits of male and female bodies. The limits are experienced as losses that are reflected in the concept of castration anxiety, with girls' anxiety being about loss of masculinity, and boys' anxiety being about loss of femininity. At first in the differentiation process, femaleness and maleness are viewed in the context of the child's own body, and then this is replaced by a complementary view that acknowledges gendered body boundaries and capacities.

As part of the oedipal phase there is a masculine stage in girls, as well as a feminine stage in boys, but it is part of the differentiation process in which there is a conflict regarding the "lost" sex characteristics of the body that are overvalued so that there is a temporary retention of alternative male and female identities. Then there is a gradual recognition of inappropriate gender identities and identification with appropriate gender identities. The second part of the oedipal phase involves a recategorization of parents in terms of genital and interpersonal masculinity and femininity. The parents become models for maleness and femaleness as external objects used to test developing subjective conceptions of being a female or a male. Rivalry and identification with the same-sex parents occur for both girls and boys, with rivalry as an opportunity for separateness. For girls the identification with the mother poses some threat to their autonomy, so it is suggested that they ultimately form a secondary identification that retains the idea of both mother and daughter being women, but allows the daughter her individuality. The cross-sex relation with father seems primarily a matter of identifying with the model of the mother as a woman rather than being motivated by sexual desire. Biological contributions to gender identity, to gender differences, and to oedipal and pre-oedipal same-sex and cross-sex relations are considered minimal.

Limitations of the differentiation model include a narrow, relatively pathological view of narcissism, a delayed timetable for self-development relative to current evidence for self- and object-differentiation, limited motivational power for the establishment of identifications, pathologizing homosexuality and bisexuality as permanent sexual preferences, and a lack of appropriate integration of biological and socializing forces in the formation of gender identity. Added to these are the strong entanglement of femininity and motherhood that Parker (1995) has noted as a problem in effectively understanding femininity. At the same time, the differentiation model illustrates the powerful role of identification in relationships that can be found in the reformulations of feminine development by Chodorow (1989) and Benjamin (1988). Also, although depicting narcissism as a state of selfness that must be given up, at the same time the work of Fast (1989) emphasizes a personal perspective in its concern with the subjective interpretation of the phenomena of gender differentiation. Essentially a reinterpretation of preoedipal and oedipal stages that does not dispute the importance of recognition of genital differences, or the existence of penis envy and castration anxiety, it reinterprets these experiences in social terms. Without clearly depicting the model as relational, it moves significantly in the relational direction that is articulated by Chodorow (1989). There is a marked trend toward understanding the interaction of the social roles and the psychology of women as contrasted with viewing women's psychology as primarily a reflection of biological forces.

Earlier Horney (1933) had rejected the belief that penis envy and the castration complex are parts of normal female development. She asserted that many of the apparent characteristics of that time, such as masochism and passive narcissistic inclinations, were functions of a patriarchal society. Also, Miller (1973) challenged masochism, penis envy, and passivity as being innate characteristics of women.

Connectedness

Jordan (1997a) describes the person as having a basic need for connection to others, which in its best form is characterized by mutual relatedness. The concepts of the self, the other, and having relationships are interconnected. The self exists in the context of relatedness, facilitated by empathy, a capacity to form gratifying attachments which leads to creative action, clarity, and a sense of confidence. Gender differences occur where males are socialized toward a power-dominance selfhood experience which emphasizes differences between the self and others. In contrast females learn to have a love-empathy way of being which facilitates mutuality. Gilligan (1982) has suggested that women define themselves in relations whereas men see separation as more attractive and empowering.

Although the potential and desire for relations is present from birth, socialization processes foster gendered differences affecting motives, values, organization of experience, and power. The developmental goals have been autonomy and objectivity for males, connection and empathy for females. Jordan considers the male goal a disruptive process of alienation and pathological narcissism, with the female goal of relationships and intersubjectivity far healthier because it is in accord with the human condition. The male goal has too often been considered the norm so that women were pathological if they failed to develop a separate, distinct self. However, a different developmental aim is suggested, namely involvement in empowering relationships, which is more congruent with the way women are raised.

This developmental model acknowledges that women have often been placed in situations of taking care of others from a subordinate position because of a society in which the masculine ideal has been dominant. However, what is suggested is that there is great value in emphasizing the relational capacities that are already fostered in female development as ways to have males and females both emphasize mutually empathic and empowering relationships. Pathology is viewed as being embodied in disconnections that result in non-mutual relationships.

Jordan (1997a) suggests that autonomy be replaced to reflect the reality of the relational nature of people's lives. Instead value would be given to clarity in feelings, thoughts, and actions, intentionality, creativity, and effectiveness that are powered through relationships and involve an awareness of the effect of individual actions upon others. "Being in relation" is the way that best describes a woman's sense of self. The model acknowledges personal history, coherence, continuity, initiative, responsiveness, body sensations, solitude, and the organization of experience as human qualities, but emphasizes the value of connection. Thus Jordan states: "An intrinsic interest and movement toward connection is a basic organizing and motivating force in psychological growth" (1997b, p. 51).

The most desirable relationship is one that is mutual and authentic, which includes being neither self-sacrificing or other-sacrificing. This introduces a personal perspective into the process, an evaluation of the mutuality by both parties which at some point has to be reduced to subjectivity. However, in this relational model such subjectivity is considered as continuously contextual, always in dialogue, and narcissism is considered a term for pathology, a selfishness that represents disconnection. The consistency of a relational self is questionable, however, because it does not provide sufficient room for intrapersonal dialogue, the voices of selves within the self, voices that transcend or are separate from voices of any others. The model could use some significant space for the expression of healthy narcissism, and the potential for this actually appears in a comment by Kaplan regarding engagement through difference. "There is only the particularity of each woman's life as she understands it, an experience that is fluid, complex, and multiply layered" (1997, p. 34).

The relational model is particularly useful in appreciating the value of an interest in others that is often highly developed in women. However, the model pays limited attention to intrapsychic structure, to the psychology of the individual, and to drives. Thus both desire and anger are depicted in relational terms primarily, making them reactive. Certainly this view accounts for some anger and some desire, but instinctual possibilities are unduly limited. At the same time, the work of Jordan et al. (1991) and Jordan (1997c) repeatedly describes itself as a "work in progress," so it is not designed to be a complete developmental theory of women. However, it is designed to portray the actualities and potentialities of women's relatedness, and it illustrates the differentiation of femininity. This distinctiveness is neatly exemplified in a quote from Irigaray, "Women's desire would not speak the same language as men's" (1985, p. 25).

Integration

A more complete model is suggested by Benjamin (1988, 1995a) in a combination of intersubjective and intrapsychic views as complementary. The intersubjective approach emphasizes individual development in relation, with the other as a subject as well as an object. The other is recognized as being both different from the self and similar, and there is a focus on what occurs between self and others. The self, when alone, is alone in a contextual way only, that is within the range of relational experience. This view does not contain a truly "alone self," because the self is already defined as relational, a context that exists at birth and continues throughout the life span. The view taken in this book of narcissism in contrast includes a truly separate self in that some aspects of aloneness are seen as referential only to the self. Thus a distinction is drawn between aspects of the self-representation that are based on differences and similarities to others and aspects that are based on observations of a personal self. For example, awareness of bodily sensations is a singular representation. Mental representations can and do take similar forms, such as a view of myself as floating in the air. In addition, there are moments of personal space, what could be considered dissociative states that are not reactions to others, present or past, but functions of a current state of reflective consciousness that also nurture one's mental and emotional existence. Thus the self is always both autonomous and relational, in varying degrees of each, and these states can be reactive to each other, but they do not have to be. There is a large unconscious component in the development of these independent states of being in that they often seem to just "come about," and it is probably impossible to prove that they are not reactive to some past relational stimulus, but they do not feel reactive. They feel owned, singular, and unique.

Benjamin (1988) accounts for some of this way of conceptualizing in her view of the intrapsychic, where the individual is seen as a separate entity with a complex internal structure of fantasies and feelings, a world of the dynamic unconscious. This is private mental space, but it becomes relational as part of the complementary process that makes up the self as having inner and outer related worlds. These are brought together by recognition which is seen as essential for establishing the feeling of the self as an agent. Benjamin acknowledges that not all actions are motivated by recognition, but emphasizes the necessity of recognition for the establishment and continuation of both a sense of mastery and of pleasure. She suggests that the ideal is mutual recognition, recognizing and being recognized by the other, with this recognition a basic developmental goal that complements separation so that there is both balance and a tension. This is a considerably broader view than the relational-connection perspective in that it adds an interpersonal view without subtracting the intrapsychic one.

A basic conflict is present between self-assertion and dependence. Establishing the self involves recognizing the other, but in this process of differentiation each state threatens the other, so there is a continual tension requiring balance, namely intersubjectivity. The relationship between self and other is an ongoing exchange of control, starting in infancy with an interest in the outside alternating with internal absorption, followed by shifts between attunement and separation. The conflicts that occur between togetherness and separateness are frequent and result in temporary polarizations, that, when not resolved in terms of returning to a balance, become states of domination.

The process of differentiation is started with complementary relationships where the parents, particularly the mother as the most frequent primary caretaker, provide nurturing experiences. These are designed to prepare for intersubjective sharing with mutual recognition, but complementarity may actually remain the primary mode of relatedness. The latter will happen if there is not a balanced pattern of destruction and survival, a setting of limits that allows for an appropriate amount of assertion as well as restriction. What is "appropriate" is a subjective concept, measured narcissistically from the perspective of the child, as well as from the parent's perspectives, but that feature is not emphasized in the theory. Instead the points are made that where destruction is commonplace, the child's sadism predominates, whereas when the survival of the other overwhelms the possibility of destruction, masochism is the more prevalent style. In either situation, a complementary domination appears rather than emotional recognition.

The sadistic style is generally attributed to males, and is partially a result of social learning. However, the psychological readiness for accepting such a style is viewed as a result of the boy's need to give up his original identification with the mother. Gender identity is established by detaching and distancing from the mother, objectifying her, and defending against the loss of individuality that identification is fantasied as bringing about by changing the early dependency into control by the boy/man. The mother's independent subjectivity is negated as she becomes the object to control.

This view tends to view identification as a total merger, or at least to view the child's fantasy about it as one of "being" the other, but this may not be the case. It is more probable that the differentiation process as it involves distinction requires adaptive defenses in the establishment of identity. The assertion of one's will has already been noted in the destruction-survival process. The subjectivity of satisfaction emphasizes different possibilities, and trying to control the other person is clearly one of them. In the case of the mother, and of women, it is not possible for the boy to turn the mother into a male, nor is it feasible for the boy to be female, so the distinction between the boy and the mother is emphasized in a fundamental way that is not needed with the father or other males. However, the desire for controlling others is not limited to the mother, but anxiety about being too much like her, as well as a growing awareness of male physical strength relative to women, all support an interest in the social role of controlling women which in turn is reinforced by the willingness of women to follow the social stereotype.

Benjamin attributes that willingness to a female acceptance of a lack of subjectivity where a women lacks recognition yet gives it. Thus the male denies the subjectivity of the other, but the female denies her subjective self. This method of establishing identity is viewed as flowing from the retention of identification with a mother who has emphasized merger rather than individuality. There is a fear of separation that results in the daughter's submission to her mother's wishes, which are exemplified in the mother's own limited ability to express desire and agency. Assertion of independence by the girl is limited by the belief that this will destroy the mother and in turn the self as shaped by identification with the mother, so masochism becomes a defensive strategy of adaptation which is in turn reinforced by social constructs of femininity.

There are a number of possible reservations about this approach. One is that the mother is not such a model of submission herself, which has become more frequent in contemporary society, and if that were the case, the girl's identification with masochism would not be likely. Another is that although a masochistic attitude toward a powerful nurturing mother could prevail, that would not have to carry over to a woman's attitude toward men unless the mother's power includes an ability to control the father, thus offering her daughter a model of dominance over men. Also, identification is being used as a fantasy of merged identity that is now based on gender likeness, while at the same time the processes of differentiation would suggest more selective identifications, including reaction formations regarding unwanted aspects of the mother. Benjamin is aware that this is only one possibility, and that there are exceptions, but her point is that explorations of cultural stereotypes such as dominant males and submissive females lies in more than social learning, or the concept of male and female "natures." She states, "But, in fact, women are not the embodiment of nature, although they have long been captives of that metaphor" (1988, p. 80).

Another way to conceptualize the masochistic interests of women is that they represent subjective appraisals of what will bring the greatest   self-satisfaction   within   the   existing   environmental circumstances. Thus, a significant amount of identifying with the mother as a model of what women do, and therefore what the girl can expect for herself, will indeed take place, but it is open to a large variety of ways in which mothers display their roles. As a result, submission may be more apparent than real, for both male and female children will develop ways to try to ensure that their needs for both dependency and assertion are satisfied. Also, a different use of the body is suggested, namely that as males gain awareness of their physical strength relative to women, females realize their relative limitations in strength. This does not make men healthier, smarter, or psychologically stronger, but they are often bigger, represented in the phallus. The symbolism of phallic power carries an inescapable logic that men usually can physically dominate women, a fact that both boys and girls learn and consider in their development of gendered attitudes. The awareness of the potential domination by gender is a significant factor in dominant-submissive complementarity.

At the same time, there is a fascination with the role of the other, noted by Benjamin in regard to sadomasochism where the patterns of domination and submission by gender are often reversed. In essence, it can be satisfying for *both* males and females to submit or to dominate. Also, in the social order there are areas of female domination and male submission, but it is possible to argue that these are essentially ceded by males in service of efficiency, as for example, child care. In essence what has prevailed is the symbolism of physical prowess, the more powerful phallic male that is feared by women, and the ideal of an individuality that is denied to women because it eradicates the need for others which is considered integral to women's nurturing selves. In contrast, Benjamin poses the possibility of balancing the recognition of other's needs with self-assertion. Such a balance actually represents the choices of narcissism, the selective application of one's own perspectives. Although Benjamin does not refer to such choices as narcissistic, she does emphasize an ongoing tension between assertion and recognition which frequently breaks down into one-dimensionality that in terms of narcissism could be considered pathological, with the return to healthy narcissism resting on the return of a dialectic tension.

Femininity has often been construed as sexual passivity, with the woman as the object of desire whose own desire is restricted to being desired. This is seen as a function of maternal identification, where the father is the object of desire, epitomized in penis envy. The girl seeks the father to get a penis, which becomes the symbol for power, desire, and freedom. However, it is not the phallus itself that is so desired, but the person of the father. Thus penis envy can be seen as a symbolic way for the girl to identify with her father as a path to autonomy that may often be limited by maternal identification.

The girl's identification with her father is particularly useful when the mother does not restrict separation, but if the mother is not operating as a subject herself, despite controlling her daughter, the identification is colored by the inequality of the parents to the point that a split is fostered in the daughter between sexuality and individuation. For both boys and girls, the father serves the role of the "other" who represents the outside world. It is not necessary that the representative be the father, but this has usually been the family situation, namely mother as representative of the "at home" world in contrast to father for the outside, or "real" world. Although the role of women as part of that real world has markedly increased, the home caretaking role has not seen a proportionate decrease. Even where child care is used extensively, the caretakers are most often women. Thus the gendering of roles, namely mothering and fathering, continues, which keeps penis envy viable as representing agency and desire embodied in the father as a wished for ideal. If the gender of the roles was switched through a change in function or family structure, or the roles were truly equalized, then this view of penis envy would need to be altered.

Benjamin postulates that the love for the father, termed identificatory love, provides a resolution for rapprochement where the child has developed ambivalence regarding dependence and separation. The awareness of the child's limits for independence threaten narcissism, and self-esteem is then repaired through identification with the father who can recognize the child's growing desire, namely locating the child as a subject. Thus the sense of agency is strongly connected at this time of life with the recognition of desire, and at this time there is also an increased awareness of the differences between mother and father symbolically represented as distinctions between dependence and independence. That distinction has actually been preceded by examples of gendered differences, such as modes of playing with the child that provide a foundation for considering the father as the existing other and the mother as the holding nurturer.

The father is more likely to accept the boy's identificatory love and support independence for the boy, which is also reinforced by the mother's greater willingness to decrease the boy's identification with her. Thus boys are characteristically moved towards autonomy by both parents. In contrast, the mother tends to maintain the girl's identification with her, being more ambivalent about her daughter's separation, and the father tends to be ambivalent about his daughter's identificatory love. Although this type of love is not to be equated with oedipal desire, it is probable that a combination of superego parental conceptions engender gendered reactions that prevent the mother and father from more effective refinements of identificatory love. As a result there is a devaluation of women for boys that accompanies the boy's paternal identification, and there is an inhibition of desire for girls in the father's ambivalent reaction to their identification with him.

Benjamin suggests that the father's disidentification from his mother accompanied by ongoing needs to differentiate from women limit his recognition of his daughter, and in turn restrict the girl's identification with the father either as a way to mitigate dependency or to establish a separate self. Thus in the rapprochement phase the girl is pushed back to the mother and gives up her desire, instead assuming a more submissive approach in idealizing a man who would have both desire and power. The identificatory love is the basis for heterosexual oedipal love. The realization of the lack of recognition via identification with the father motivates a desire to posses the father, but this desire is often colored by both submission and envy. In addition, the girl's desire is also limited by the frequent lack of a mother who can be perceived as a sexual agent with her own desire.

Both parents could be separation and attachment objects and subjects for boys and girls, but generally they are more distinctive so that the children become gender limited in their possible use of identifications. These identifications are being attempted in the preoedipal period when the process is relatively fluid and overinclusive (Fast, 1984) so that identifications are not viewed by the child as requiring gender polarity. The continued fluidity of identifications, or selective identification, is in fact possible and useful throughout life, particularly as a way to understand others as well as the self. However, it is often restricted by parents and defended against by their children as adults because it is seen as a threat to both gender identity and gender role identity.

The failure of identificatory love for girls enhances the possibility of masochistic approaches which both serve as attempts to overcome dependency and to submit. Identificatory love is distorted into submission, which is facilitated by the mother's lack of subjectivity. Thus although connection theory emphasizes the mother's nurturance, there is often an ambivalence in which subjectivity and femininity are not synthesized. Although the boy has a greater possibility of access to the father's identificatory love, it is tinged by the need to distance from and devalue women, a tendency that is unwittingly reinforced by the boy's mother moving him away from identificatory love with her. Furthermore, Benjamin points out that the culture reinforces the father, and thus males, as the idealized symbols of power and desire, leaving women to struggle with their own potential for desire, and leaving men as unwilling to trade the favored position of greater autonomy for the possible satisfaction of mutual recognition. Such a gendered division is being challenged, particularly in terms of its fundamental "naturalness," as well as the interpretation of clinical observations, such as penis envy. In this challenge it is useful to return to the personal perspective of narcissism as a way to understand both acceptance and revolt against current structures of femininity and masculinity.

Although Benjamin does not use the concept of narcissism in this way, she does provide an understanding of how the personal perspective can work. She acknowledges the symbolism of phallic power and desire, and then considers alternatives. A possibility is to put female organs on the same representational level as male organs, a possibility that would be initiated by the correct knowledge of female genitals in childhood which would include the awareness of female desire with its own special qualities. While this knowledge and awareness is certainly useful, women's bodies are already idealized in the culture, although as objects of desire. The representation of women is the issue, and maternal representation has been desexualized as well as feared, and in turn devalued. In essence, Benjamin points out that for the most part it is a phallic representational world, and that women's desire will not come into its own by trying to turn it into a vaginal symbolic world. Instead she suggests a recognition of intersubjective experience that has been neglected in favor of the intrapsychic. The intersubjective stresses the recognition of the other as the major component of differentiation, as opposed to separateness of the self. Erotic union, expression of sexual desire, then involves mutual recognition with pleasure given and gotten with and in the other. Furthermore, the intersubjective desire is expressed as spatial representation, with inner space as active receptivity and self-exploration. Women's desire becomes the desire to be known both via having her own space that can be without intrusion, or can be penetrated. The sexual self can be represented by the body's entire sensual possibilities, an avenue open to men as well. Thus coexistence of intrapsychic and intersubjective sexualities is being proposed, rather than glorifying one mode of expression.

> The relationship itself, ... the exchange of gestures conveying attunement, and not the organ, serves to focus women's pleasure and contain their anxiety. Women make use of the space in-between that is created by shared feeling and discovery. The dance of mutual recognition, the meeting of separate selves, is the context for their desire (1988, p. 130).

The oedipal situation is also subject to reinterpretation, so that it is one step in development that builds upon preoedipal identification and is open to subsequent levels of integration. It is a time of increased desire for the other, a different erotic love than identificatory love, and it is a time for increased awareness of differentiation in which males and females both come to a resolution of differences instead of stressing polarities. The result provides for mutual recognition and generalized gender identifications. It is understood however, that recognition is not always operating, that tension gives way to unequal complementarity or essentially domination, but what is possible is the restoration of tension by dealing with contradictions within the self. However, it must be noted that there has to be a desire to do this, which returns us to the power of narcissism. The personal perspective of what is feminine, of what is satisfactory to the girl/woman, is the ultimate motivator. The model of duality and submission has been the one generally offered, but that is shifting, and a model that includes both the intrapsychic and intersubjective dimensions is a considerable step towards a better understanding of femininity. Thus it is possible to work with the vagueness of desire as depicted in the intersubjective model, to question the force of recognition, to wonder whether the intrapsychic has to be viewed as so exclusionary, in essence to argue with aspects of Benjamin's approach and still appreciate the significance of her reconceptualization of the roles and psychic developments of both women and men. In her valuation of the need for recognition there is a congruence with a conception of narcissism that emphasizes the subjectivity of interaction. Her concern is with intersubjectivity, and the tension of relating to the self and the other, but in calling for recognition of the other as a subject rather than just an object, the need of the subject is the point of origin. The desire for recognition, as well as other desires, are part of a subjective viewpoint which involves movement between the degree to which one recognizes another as a subject and in turn gives up some of one's own subjectivity, and the degree to which the other is an object who recognizes the self. The specifics of this interplay are worked out between the people involved, so there is mutuality, but it is an asymmetrical mutuality in that the subjects view themselves as more or less attuned and satisfied. However, it is not possible for one subject to completely know the other, or given the power of the unconscious, for the self to be completely known. There is always a mix of private and social, hidden and exposed, so therefore the "tension" in recognition of the self, of the other, or by the self and by the other. Narcissism is construed here as organizing, distributing, and balancing this tension.

The progression of healthy narcissism in the formation of a feminine identity includes a subjective congruence between behavior and anatomy. The latter provides a variety of characteristics that are potentials for femininity, with traditional and nontraditional forms of using these potentials. The passage of time has played a role in the formation of adaptation, such as the woman breast feeding the child or using mutual cueing to facilitate development. Part of that adaptation has been developing a fit between the self of the woman with motivations such as libido and aggression, separation and connection, and a patriarchal society in which men hold more of the power and thus restrict the potential of women. This power originates in physical strength and subsequent corresponding division of labor that fostered a warrior-nurturer dichotomy. In contemporary societies, most such divisions are outmoded, but the balance of power has not been shifted to the point of equality. Rules of force, whether diplomatic, economic, or the size of one's army, tend to govern most of the world so that androcentric societies remain the norm. The duality of human nature, constructive and destructive, is a foundation for conflict and tension, and women are less privileged than men in their ability to assert their motivations. However, as is the case with men, narcissism represents their personal balancing act. Although it at the moment seems difficult to prove that males or females are innately motivated primarily in a drive (libido and aggression) or a relational mode, or even some other superordinate mode, and until otherwise established it appears prudent to postulate a variety of major motivations, there has been some tendency to assume that women are innately more social, that this in turn is restricted by men who overvalue autonomy and have made it the norm, and that a return to women's nature is more desirable. However, it is hypothesized here that men and women enter into the world with the same duality of conflicting tendencies, but male power has prevailed, primarily as a result of pathological narcissism that dictates the potentialities of phallic power. Thus women have to struggle with the oppression of gender, and have to do more to bring about gender balance in regard to desire and its satisfaction. As Jessica Benjamin noted in 1988, "...how much the reality of women's condition differs from what we, in our minds, have long since determined it should be. Even the more modest demands for equality that we take for granted have not been realized" (p. 87).

Approximately 12 years later, Benjamin's comments remain true. This society may be committed by law and spirit to equal opportunities for women and men, but such an approach threatens the established order for both men and women. Thus the girl of the present continues to be born into an androcentric society where it often seems easier for her to follow a model of traditional femininity which emphasizes nurturance and selective agency, such as some types of income-producing work.

Of course this does not mean that the girl will automatically fall into line, or that she should. Her personal perspective will be based on what feels best for her. Nurturance may not suit her, anatomy and physiology may not cooperate in her being the stereotyped female. Also, the assumption of a female role involves a variety of partial identifications derived from parents and other significant people who appear to the child to have appealing attributes, and in this regard the identificatory figures themselves may be offering different values that stress a greater potential for women than was presented in past generations. Also, it is not the literal mother or father that has to be identified with, although incorporation and introjection at times can feel to the child as though she is the other person, but ultimately it is the symbolism of the other that represents the identification that can be facilitated and reinforced through mirroring, idealizing, recognition, and identificatory love. Thus the girl child can assume whatever qualities she desires, such as agency, but with the differentiation that she is an agentic female. This is in accord with the early establishment of gender differentiation and core gender identity and would only be missing or a source of conflict in the small number of people who actually want to be anatomically different. The core gender identity is not to be equated with gender role identity, so that is possible to identify the self as female and favor "masculine" modes of being, or to choose a same-sex sexual partner.

The process of differentiation will begin at birth, and the girl will repeatedly be told she is like the mother and different from the father in gendered terms. Both girls and boys may also be told they are like the opposite sex parent in various ways, but it will usually be made clear that their gender is unaffected by such likenesses. Actually, parents and families vary in the degree to which they foster gendered identification, so qualities possessed by either or both parents can become part of a female identification. The girl tests out what works for her and tries to put that into effect. Of course parents and others will usually try to move the girl in a direction they consider feminine, but that does not mean she has to follow their urgings. She does, however, need to understand what girls and men usually do in this society, and be aware that there are consequences to doing the unusual.

The development of femininity (and masculinity) must provide for an exploration of gender role identities that includes a variety of sexual orientations and preferences, as well as degrees of ambivalence, without resorting to a heterosexual triadic resolution as the healthy norm. As Kubie asked in 1974, why should ambivalence be considered universal, except in regard to gender. Many people who ostensibly demonstrate heterosexual orientations have limited success with such focusing of their desire as well as its enactment. In fact, any gender role identity and its specific behaviors and fantasies may be symptomatic and defensive, but only a relatively small number of sexual enactments qualify as categorically pathological. Same-sex erotic preference is not one of the few, yet psychoanalytic developmental theories usually fail to explain it as part of a normal developmental line that can have a viable outcome.

Whether any sexuality is a biologically-rooted preference or a learned disposition in terms of object choice remains a disputed matter (Herron & Herron, 1996). Let us hypothesize that erotic preferences are combinations of physical predispositions and psychological experiences that operate in a society that is relatively homophobic and that finds it expedient for most people to enact heterosexuality and produce triadic gendered families. Clearly the degree of family pathology that exists illustrates that approach is no guarantee of health due to its social endorsement. Other possibilities, while socially more complicated, have viability and have to be understood as potential developmental pathways that also need normative explanations. This point was made in the previous chapter on masculine development, and proposals in this regard have been made by a number of authors (Friedman, 1986; Isay, 1989;

Lewes, 1995), but have not met with general acceptance in analytic theory. The problem is apparent in regard to lesbian development as well (Burch, 1992, 1993), so that what is needed is a developmental theory that does not depend on pathology to explain anything other than heterosexuality, and that also takes into account the multiplicities of relationships, namely different types and degrees of sexualities.

In suggesting that homosexuality can be seen as a pathway for optimal development for some individuals, Burch emphasizes the importance of a personal perspective, namely what is the best fit for a particular person, which is in accord with narcissism as an organizing principle. "We require a wider view of human sexual development, one that considers these strategic resolutions as a triumph of the psyche's creative potential rather than dismissing them as pathology" (1993, p. 98).

Women's sexual development in general has traditionally been pathologized to the extent that psychoanalytic theory emphasized negation of personal sexuality and acceptance of inferiority relative to the phallic world dominated by males. The association of penis and power that is vested in masculinity and that tends to include physical strength is only one part of masculinity. The obviousness of the male genitals also point to their vulnerability, and males are noticeably vulnerable to physical attack and pain in the genital area. Furthermore, women have considerable physical strength and endurance, generally displaying it in different ways than men, such as childbearing, but women are certainly kept in touch with their bodily sensations, for example in the menstrual cycle. Thus it is important to take into account body awareness in the development of femininity. Past psychoanalytic theory has emphasized what women did not have, namely the penis, but Mayer (1995) has pointed out that female gender identity starts with an awareness of the girl's body as it is, "a state of having something distinctive" (p. 18).

The work of De Marneffe (1997) indicates that at approximately 22 months girls have an awareness of their genitals and are pleased with them, which in turn indicates a mental representation of genital femininity. Mayer (1995) and Tyson (1994) link this genital representation to the concept of primary femininity (Stoller, 1977), an identity that involves the girl's sense of her female body that develops in the preoedipal period prior to having penis envy (Elise, 1997). A further distinction is suggested here because of the implication that femininity could be innate and that such a view would make the learned part of femininity (which appears to be the major part) insignificant. Elise points out that "primary" currently is employed to describe a sense of self that is bodily derived. It is important to note that although this is usually symbolized through the genitals, and genital differences, the entire body schema is a more accurate portrayal. Different body specifics come into play at different phases of life. For example, for the infant boy to be mirrored as a "big boy" usually has only little to do with the size, or even the existence, of his penis, but more to do with his height and weight. Similarly, for the infant girl to be mirrored as a "pretty girl" is not dependent mainly on her genitals, but other bodily features. Of course "big" and "pretty" are gendered cultural values, but they also have observable referents, and as such are part of the self-representation.

Elise (1997) also points out that femininity is used in two different ways that are not really interchangeable, although they are certainly related, The first is to describe a sense of self derived from being biologically female, and the second is a learned experience that becomes internalized. To clarify this distinction, Elise suggests using "primary sense of femaleness" to depict the early mental representations of the body, and to separate this from femininity, which accompanies the former only in varying degrees. Thus the various characteristics of femininity are not essential to being a woman, although the ways of "being feminine" are conventionally known. As with masculinity, some characteristics of femininity are useful and appealing, others harmful but appealing, and some are not appealing. Also, some are attainable by most women, and some are attainable only by a few. Elise (1997) makes the point that there is not always congruence with femaleness, femininity, and sexual orientation.

Being a female is one part of a personal identity whose form beyond the anatomy is environmentally shaped, yet interactive given the feelings of each individual female. Thus a woman can feel whatever way she wants about her genitals, including penis envy, but it is factual that the existence of her genitals provides her with specific potentials for pleasure, behavior, and fantasy, with pleasurable sensations beginning early in life. How sexuality, femininity, and body parts will coalesce and be used is going to be a matter of personal style. The function and symbolism of the body have played a part in the process of identification. Women's sexual anatomy is treated ambivalently in an androcentric culture. The power to have a baby is respected and envied, but this is woman as the powerful mother in comparison to the man as always powerful because he has a penis. Actually the genitals of both genders have power in the performance of a sexual function with the possibility of reproduction, but they are not guarantees of other powers or strengths. Actually being smart and creative are better prognostic signs for extensive power. However, the phallic bias needs to be addressed for women because both genders continue to be in relative conformity to it, and it is particularly restrictive for women. At the same time, the cultural mode is a complex issue that in its asymmetry holds certain strong appeals to each gender. For example, the powerful male can be invoked as a security for the female to whom he is committed as a protector, just as the nurturing woman is reassuring for the self-esteem of the male when his power is threatened. While the reality of these images is far from universal, they happen enough to often outweigh the appeal of a more significant change in gender opportunities and desires.

Ideals remain elusive and results are often confusing in terms of satisfactions, but personalizing the gender issue would be a help. This means paying more attention in the developmental process to what individuals want, given in this case their primary femaleness and their variety of options regarding gender role identities. The identification with femininity is fostered in the degree of gender differentiation that is appropriate to the society. It is not necessary that the girl be disconnected from either her mother or her father, or whomever the significant caretaker is, as long as there are boundaries that keep separation and connection in a working alliance and enable the establishment and enjoyment of these states with others beyond the family and with and for the self.

The initial differentiation between the infant and the mother is such that there can be the coexistence of ideas of being and not being the mother, as well as being and not being other significant figures. Included in this process are part-object distinctions and mergers as well. As differentiation increases a sense of distinctiveness and wholeness accompanies a sense of connection. Connections with others are reshaped around both anatomy and function. The girl is taught and learns that she is supposed to be more similar to her mother than to her father. The similarity is basically biological, but customarily the parents and society have added specific qualities to the anatomical likeness and created a constellation of traits and behaviors that are deemed feminine. Thus what it means to be feminine becomes more of a social construction than inherent (Elise, 1997; Mayer, 1995; Tyson, 1994).

The specifics of this femininity have been developed historically over time in response to various personal environmentally adaptive needs, but they are open to change. As noted in regard to masculinity, such changes occur slowly because of the attractions of the existing power from psychological, evolutionary, and social perspectives. For example, Elise comments: "With both mother and daughter residing in a patriarchal culture, female difficulties, including a sense of inadequacy, deprivation, and unresolved anger, may persist" (1997, p. 514).

The shaping of identity in regard to being female does mean that the girl, as the boy, gives up the idea of unlimited gender potentials. This is a time that has been characterized as one of overinclusiveness (Elise, 1997; Fast, 1984) that is a product of a narcissistic sense of omnipotence that will be followed by a sense of loss or damage when the limits are discovered. However, a number of possibilities exist in this state, all of which are based on limited knowledge of being male or female and what males and females can or cannot do. Not knowing the actuality of one's potential is not equivalent to assuming that one can do anything that another person can do. At first the child lacks knowledge of its powers, so the child fantasizes about them, but not necessarily in an exclusively omnipotent manner. This also means that the gaining of knowledge is not always about what one cannot do, but also is about what one can do that may have previously been an unknown possibility. Elise (1997) begins an elaboration of the gender differentiation model when she points out there is a time when the self-representation contains both a lack of knowledge of gender limits as well as an unawareness of the existing effects of such limits.

She suggests that the girl and boy both have fantasies of bisexual completeness, but the specifics of the fantasy have a gender differentiation due to the person's particular anatomy, physiology, and caretaking experiences. This is depicted as an unlimited gender potential categorized as bisexuality, but it seems more accurate to describe it as a changing, and in that sense, unknown sexual potential that is essentially pansexual. It may be quite limited, and more person-specific than gender specific, although it is certainly linked to gender identity. In contrast is may be very expansive, depending on one's fantasies and knowledge. Also, as Elise points out in regard to bisexuality, a primary sense of femaleness, or maleness, can accompany the bisexuality. This view can be expanded to include a recognition of gender identity without being tied to object choice limitations. In essence the basic limitations are anatomical (what one's body can do) and psychic (the representation of desire), so that gender role identity is very much a narcissistic choice, being who the person wants to be.

Mayer (1995) describes femininity as a state of having something that is distinctive, but describes an accompanying feature of female genital anxiety. This anxiety refers to the loss of female capacities. Both girls and boys are conceptualized as having initial self-representations of their bodies as they are, followed by perceptions of difference and then concern about what may be missing. Part of that concern for girls includes a phallic castration complex, namely the fantasy of a lost penis, a fear that is both more obvious and common in boys (Elise, 1997). Mayer (1995) suggests that when depression is the major compromise formation for a woman, it is related primarily to the phallic castration anxiety. Depression is a defensive strategy that is concerned with a wish to alter the past which is seen as negative. Thus the focus would be on undoing the beginning fact of being a woman. The danger has happened, with depression as the defensive motive in line with a fantasy that the girl was turned into a woman by having lost the penis. In this case there are symptoms of deficiency and inadequacy. However, these same symptoms may indeed occur in anxiety where the conflict is considered to be over primary femininity where danger is now anticipated, the female genital is valued, and there is a fear that it will be damaged in some way.

Mayer (1995) describes the anxiety defense configuration as primary femininity, but both affect-defense approaches appear to be part of the concept of female genital anxiety, one emphasizing the possibility of damage to what exists, the other of damage to what is imagined to have been. Thus this concept of primary femininity appears significantly different from what is usually depicted as primary femininity, although it does make the major point noted by Tyson (1994) and Elise (1997) that girls begin with a self-representation of what they have, rather than focusing on what they may appear to be missing. What these three contemporary authors emphasize, although in varying degrees with Elise being the strongest about it, is that women's problems have much more to do with being women than not being men. In essence, women are defining themselves, and do so from birth on, primarily in terms of what it means to be a female, as contrasted with a more traditional view of self-definition based on what it means not to be a male. For each gender, then, that gender is the major referent in normal development, rather than masculinity operating as a practical norm. Tyson and Mayer tend however to vest concepts such as penis envy and castration anxiety with more significance than does Elise, as well as making female development more intrapsychic than interpersonal, intersubjective, and cultural. Thus the reconceptualizations by Elise are more reflective of relational contemporary theorists of feminine development, such as Benjamin (1995a) and Jordan (1997c).

The shaping of identity in regard to being a female does mean that the girl loses the possibility of looking like and being a father. Although such an identity is an anatomical illogicality that is contradicted by her designation from birth as a girl, it can be considered a loss in a patriarchal culture. However, as Tyson (1994) points out, given the anatomical similarity with the girl's usual first object, her mother, a sense of body integrity is probably more fixed than it is for boys, thus mitigating a sense of loss when anatomical differences are noticed. More of a force than anatomy is the attitude of the parents, particularly the mother, in fostering a feminine identity (Bernstein, 1983; Elise, 1997). In fact, the negative evaluation of many aspects of femininity in the culture have been internalized by caretakers and in turn the daughters.

> ...certain difficulties in female development may stem in significant part from the cultural devaluation of woman, the impact of which the mother may have experienced with her own mother and which in various ways may filter into her interaction with her daughter (Elise, 1997, p. 509).

The parents play a key role in forming the transitions in both the type of identifications that are being fostered and the meaning of these identifications in terms of gender role identity, particularly object choice. Close relationships with both parents will ideally be fostered from birth so that the infant can feel strongly connected to the qualities of each parent. The parents have the opportunities to instill pride in the child's gender identity, to indicate the paths usually taken in the culture, as well as other options, and the problems associated with different manifestations of gender role identity. What the girl becoming woman makes of all this is where narcissism enters.

The set of rules or customs by which women are to function were always subjectively experienced and in turn defined, but nature was given more of a role than nurture in the apparent feminine role. The range of approved narcissistic possibilities has been relatively limited. Sexual preference/orientation was to be heterosexual, and role behaviors such as nurturance, suffering, and passivity were considered normative expectations for women. Deviations, such as lesbianism, assertiveness, and success were met with social disapproval. Women who failed to met gender role goals were expected to keep trying and accept an accompanying "gender strain."

Actually, instead of being inherent the major portion of the content of femininity was learned from anatomical possibilities, from caretakers, and from society. A personal perspective that differed from what was expected was not reinforced, or it was undermined, or it was defended against by parents as well as by the developing female, creating a conflict for anyone outside the norm. The description by Mayer (1995) of women defending against the depression of feeling ineffective as well as defending against the anxiety of ambition exemplify typical results of struggling with narcissism. The narcissistic ego ideal for many women was, and still remains, the functional ideal of a patriarchal society. Despite shifts in society so that role possibilities and images have indeed expanded for women, Elise notes that "femininity is still a compromised identity for many" (1997, p. 508).

In addition to anatomical and biological predisposition, the idea of identifying with the mother has always been a major conception in explaining the acquisition of a female identity. However, that requires several qualifications. A certain amount of disidentification or partial identifications are needed for sufficient autonomy to occur, and mothers have traditionally been more facilitory of these "moments of separation" for boys than for girls. Identification with the father is also important in regard to confirmation of the girl's femininity, but that tends to be restricted both by fathers themselves, who grant recognition more readily to their sons, as well as by mothers who tend to be the gatekeepers for girls' access to their fathers as well as being image makers of the fathers. In addition, what the mother offers as a role model often will not conform to what the daughter finds most appealing. For example, Campbell (1993) points out that mothers often promote the idea that for their daughters to establish and sustain relationships the girls must restrict their aggression, and Elise (1991) has also found mothers discouraging girls from expressing aggression.

In the developmental process there appears to be limited, partial, and shifting identifications with parental figures and significant others which find a fit within the individual and which subsequently come together into an identity that includes a gender role. The components of that identity are a function of narcissism as a personal perspective on developmental events. Narcissism is subject to the major motivations suggested in pscyhoanalytic theories, such as pleasure, safety, approval, love, attachment, contact, recognition, creativity, cohesion, and integrity. There is also an increasing awareness of a need to act to get what one desires, and an awareness of "girlness" that is akin to "relatedness" in the integration of an identity. The girl-woman is partially identified by her body, and in that sense can most easily identify with her mother and other females in the framework of a primary femaleness. Her feelings about the identification will vary in terms of the degree of acceptance and pleasure in having a female body and the use she makes of it, but unless she changes the anatomy of her gender, which happens in only a small number of women, she will try to make the most adaptive use of it. What is viewed by each person as "most adaptive" is a matter of the personal perspective, namely the woman's narcissism.

Beyond anatomy the very substantial rest of the female identity provides more options for expression, although there are social superego-type boundaries involved that get flexed or broken only at some affective cost. Sharing certain aspects of early child-rearing for example is behavior that some women will resist because they see no personal advantage to doing it. At the same time the idea that because one is female means one must be the primary nurturer can feel a burden that some women would prefer not to have. The existence of "gender strain" in trying to fulfill the female gender role emphasizes the narcissistic conflict. Narcissism contains the message of getting your needs met, but the needs often become conflictual. Healthy female narcissism, just as healthy male narcissism, refuses the small incremental gains of momentary satisfaction in favor of a broader subjective perspective of personal integrity and respect, a feeling that is worked out in processes such as mutuality and intersubjectivity. The female world is by custom a world of putting others ahead of the self in ways that actually can be detrimental to both the self and others. As a result it takes considerable wisdom and courage to feel comfortable as a woman who actually acknowledges and respects her narcissism. Benjamin (1988) has noted the failure of psychological theories to adequately describe the independent existence of the mother, and has stressed the importance of the nurturing mother to reflect a separate subjectivity. There are of course many avenues to different types of societies, but history does argue against any of them soon becoming sufficiently egalitarian that females will be relieved of either the burdens or enjoyments of self-sacrifice. However, it is also unlikely that female agency will decrease, or that females will be encouraged to be less assertive. Just as is the case with male narcissism, female narcissism has to be opened up to more affective and behavioral possibilities. This does not mean that one quality will replace another, as for example assertion will not remove connection, nor will there be a lack of gender differentiation in the sense of using and enjoying the specialness of femaleness and maleness that is not connected to a differentiation of domination.

At present it is difficult to define femininity, the female role, or what it means to be a woman because these are all evolving issues. The threat of maternal connection as well as the need for it, and the ambivalence of paternal recognition as well as the need for that are childhood issues repeated throughout life for the woman. Any significant person, as well as the self, can be powerful as a source of love or hate. Thus the parents and society and culture have a complex interactive task of providing the individual female child with the knowledge of options and the support to take them. The best perspective is one of equal opportunity, but it is very subjective to attempt to elaborate specifics. A significant amount of literature (Benjamin, 1995a; Chodorow, 1989; Elise, 1997; Jordan, 1997c) suggests that women should have a greater sense of agency, but the autonomy implied by agency is seen by some women as opposed to a sense of valued connectedness and/or to the safety of dependency on males. Some of the traditional submissiveness is gladly given up, but some, particularly the part of being cared for, or having the status of primary nurturer, remains valued by many women. The coexistence and reformulation of the mix of, for example, self-esteem and safety, or recognizing and being recognized, are works in progress.

Thus, we come back to the idea that the female can best be aided in the development of her identity by understanding that there are in a sense no roles that have to be assumed for a person to be a female, as well as that there are adaptive consequences in choosing how to display a feminine gender role identity. In addition it is clear that characteristics such as agency and recognition are valuable narcissistic attributes for women, particularly when it comes to being a mother, a role that is likely to remain prominent in present as well as future female gender role identifications.

Mothering

The cultural connection between being a woman and being a mother is so powerful that it tends to become an equation, but such an equation is inaccurate and causes problems for women in establishing their identity. This is particularly apparent for women who are unable to give birth, or who do not wish to have a child, or have negative feelings about being a mother. Nonetheless, Finzi states: "Among the most powerful images that culture has elaborated both to represent and to govern women, is, without a doubt, that of motherhood" (1996, p. 146).

Psychoanalysis has been very much a part of this cultural construction, including the specifics of mothering that emphasize the pathology that mothers are capable of producing. "Mother-blaming" has been well documented in the psychoanalytic literature (Caplan & Hall-McCorquodale, 1985; Van Mens-Verhulst, 1994) and has been accompanied by numerous descriptions of how mothers need to behave in order to provide for the emotional health of their children. The ideal mother is primarily a nurturer who always puts her children's needs ahead of hers, and in fact appears to lack subjectivity other than an overpowering desire and will to care for her children. Negative feelings about children or mothering tend to be viewed as pathological and unacceptable, thus leaving no room for the range of feelings that mothers actually experience.

The image of the mother throughout history appears to have been a shifting one which attests to the ambivalence of mothers, although it has not usually been interpreted that way. Instead there has been a focus on social, political, economic, and religious circumstances that could be construed as affecting maternal attitudes. An example is the abandonment of babies which at certain times was accepted by society, and then changed in apparent response to a growing awareness of the value of all people to the society (Badinter, 1981). Parker (1995) makes the point that there were always different views of mothers and mothering, and that social and historical trends interact with a basically ambivalent parent-child relationship. The mother has been and continues to be viewed in a variety of inconsistent ways that have tended to deny the complexity of her subjectivity. Finzi (1996) notes the following cultural metaphors of motherhood; mother-earth, maternity as intellectual labor, maternity as creativity, and mother as goodness, and these are only some of the possibilities.

Parker (1995) points out that pregnancy itself is a contradictory situation for a woman, a wanted addition and an unwanted deprivation. The mother may feel as though she has received a gift or a burden, that she has received a welcome visitor or been violated by an intruder, that she has extended herself or that she has lost part of her personal space. There is considerable probability of repeating aspects of her own early relationship with her mother. Pregnancy offers the possibilities of reparation via identification with a loving mother as well as fears of retaliation and destruction. It is often a time of contradiction, shifting identifications with being a mother and being the mother's child, being creative and being victimized, with projection to the fetus of a variety of mixed, and at times, dichotomized feelings.

In discussing the various common maternal images, there has to be an understanding that external characteristics, such as ethnicity, socioeconomic status, and marital status, as well as how the mothering has come about, for example by sexual intercourse, adoption, or step-parenting, affect the internal life of the mother. Bell Scott et al. (1993) illustrate differences between African-American and white perceptions on motherhood, and in addition, Phoenix, Woollett, and Lloyd (1991) point out variations within categories, such as African-American women, Thus descriptions of mothering will at times appear to be generalizations that miss distinctions that are functions of external circumstances interacting with intrapsychic concerns. In such instances, reinterpretation of apparent commonalities is required. At the same time, there are relatively common conceptions of mothering that tend to have an impact on most woman who are mothers.

One major conception is the mother and child as a fused unit which is seen as the satisfaction of women's desire for connection. This desire for union, which is represented in experiences of a strong sense of harmony and oneness during infancy, is both idealized and at the same time viewed as the source of mothers being unable to facilitate separation in their children, particularly daughters. This is an ideal of complete devotion which at the same time will have to be constantly altered to account for separation desires on the child's part, so it is an unreachable ideal, essentially frustrating, Of course it also is a questionable conclusion that women want such an exclusionary relationship with their children. The mother's separateness is of major significance, as well as the relationship with a partner in the parenting process. An interest in moments of fusion, or instances of complete empathy, is different form a constant need for types of merger. Furthermore, Parker (1995) suggests that what women desire, and in turn what is also reflective of their experiences of ambivalence, are times of sharing rather than fusion.

As part of the oneness conception, mothers are viewed ideally as accepting containers of the aggression of their children rather than retaliating. However, Winnicott (1965) had taken note of the inevitability of hostile feelings in the mother, and Klein (1980) described persecutory anxiety as the mother's phantasy of being victimized by the child as well as depressive anxiety about destructive feelings towards the child. In essence, the case was made for an ambivalent mother, but not for the acceptance and use of the ambivalence. Parker (1995) suggests a spectrum of feeling from containment to abusive retaliation, but the predominance of aggression is generally limited by the mother's ability to feel for the child rather than identifying with the child's aggression. Also, a certain amount of inevitable depression associated with a sense of loss of a good internal object requires an awareness of the "normalcy" of ambivalence and the use of differentiation of the self from the child. Clearly at times the mother will feel a sense of being helpless that is experienced as quite distinct from her sense of power.

The mother is involved in an ongoing negotiation of both connection and separation. Narcissism is satisfied at different times by both possibilities, and both are also valued as well as criticized by society, as well as by the superego of the mother. The good mother nurtures properly, and that includes balancing connection and separation, but the guilt tends to be stronger in regard to the mother wanting to be a separate person in relation to her children. As a result, personal desires that would result in maternal separation, such as career, are subject to reproach as though they were motivated by wanting to neglect the child. A risk is posed to the presence of a positive internal object which supports the idea of consistency between nurturance and satisfaction of other subjective desires. Mothering can both support the presence of a good internal object and undermine it with significant moments of inadequacy. The use of the mother as an object has been noted by Winnicott, but the mother is also capable of using the baby as an object. The process of destroying the object is available to the mother as well. Samuels (1989) describes how aggressive fantasy, object destruction, is a facilitator of relating because it is tied to the knowing and using of objects, namely it is a type of connection that also highlights differentiation. Samuels (1993) has also noted that the predominant emphasis on the mother-child union neglects babies' desires to separate, mothers' individuations, and makes fathers the "necessary others," the outsiders in a sense, who force separation, which of course dichotomizes the fathers along with the mothers, when it is more likely that they are ambivalent and play multiple roles in both separation and connection.

Mothering is generally associated with a female gender role identity that is part of the attainment of gender consistency, and represents productivity or nurturing by the female. This gender consistency starts with the categorizing of people by gender and is subsequently reinforced by an awareness of the immutable aspects of gender, what one has and what one does not have. Genital awareness and an awareness of genital differences appears relatively early in development and are part of a general body outline. For the female this is usually associated with the knowledge that femininity and mothering go together, and such knowledge often includes the functions of being a mother. Although there are ideas and fantasies of overinclusion, as well as the possibilities of cross-gender preoedipal behavior, the mother is very available for identification so that the images of mothering are very much a part of a complex representation of femininity that is also attracted to personal needs that may seem at variance with being a mother. Of course many of the functions of both mothering and fathering are not categorically gender-limited, but they tend to be offered that way, particularly in regard to mothering. Nonetheless mothering as part of the expression of gender identity reflects a shifting relationship among psychic forces as well as being interactive with social expectations and social reality. In that sense it is always narcissistic with continual redoings of the needs and demands that are generated internally and externally.

The role of the mother is certainly a confusing one because the mother is asked to be strong in certain situations, and weak in others; supportive in many instances, frustrating in others to foster separation. The intertwining feminine maternal role is filled with contradictions and problems for the woman. For example, the image that mother-earth represents has a very long history (Merchant, 1980) which symbolizes a duality, earth as the nurturer, but earth as also the final recipient of the body. This metaphor puts motherhood in the domain of nature to the exclusion of individuality, and emphasizes its inevitability, a submission by the woman. The presumed naturalness can also conceal the work of productivity and the social function of maternity and child-rearing (Finzi, 1996).

The potential inevitability of motherhood is a strong factor even in the weakest of mother-daughter identifications, and usually the bond is relatively strong in promoting the narcissistic value to a woman of being a mother. Tubert (1997) has pointed out the power of the expectation that a woman will become a mother where the infertile woman appears as both uncreative and unnatural. The lure of motherhood is narcissistic fulfillment in operating in accord with the suggested essence of a woman, yet the option of any other view of femininity is foreclosed. However, there is no question that the personal perspective of most women contains a strong maternal desire that woman strive to accomplish, and often suffer narcissistic injury if they fail to become a mother.

The situation becomes further complicated once the woman is a mother because she is then relying on a number of identifications of varying degrees with significant mothering figures in her life, including the father-as-mother, but particularly her own mother, or in the case of an absent biological mother, the woman who has been the most significant mothering figure to her. She may agree with the mother who is shadowing her to the point of merger and replication, or disagree to the point of repudiation and reversal. Along with the personal identifications are desires to please, wishes for adoration, reverence, and respect, fantasies of personal fulfillment through the created children, and the specter of ambivalence that is often represented in separation-connection conflicts as mothering is in progress.

The difficulty in being a mother is described by Raphael-Leff (1991) as an ongoing tension between the woman's individuality and being a caretaker of a separate yet dependent-in-transition other person. Starting with birth, or even pregnancy, it is quite possible to feel a unity with the helplessness of what is created as well as feeling one is the powerful creator, a shifting, and at times conflicting personal perspective. The woman comes to mothering with her own narcissistic ideal of what will make her feel satisfied in mothering. For example, satisfying the child for some mothers feels powerful, but for others it is an oppressive demand that reduces the sense of self to powerlessness. Raphael-Leff (1993) describes three types of mothers, namely the Facilitator, the Regulator, and the Reciprocator. The Facilitator adapts to the baby as a way to diminish hostility on both her part and the part of the baby, whereas the Regulator keeps connection at a distance by making the infant adapt to her. Thus the former fears hostility and the latter fears intimacy whereas the Reciprocator tolerates ambivalence. Parker (1995) points out that both the Facilitator and the Regulator are attempting to take care of the child appropriately as they deem what is correct, thus emphasizing subjectivity, and this is done both for the child and to maintain their own sense of goodness, essentially demonstrating a narcissistic orientation. This is true of the Reciprocator as well, but in her case the approach is more congruent with her range of feelings and so is more likely to illustrate healthy narcissism.

Parker (1995) describes a number of other possibilities in which one side of ambivalence dominates to the point of causing a problem in the mother-child relationship and damaging the mother's self-esteem. One is where the need to control the child in a protective way causes the mother to be frustrated with the child's resistance and to hit the child. This is then followed by regret and shame at the loss of control and the hurt that she has inflicted on the child. This reaction sequence is viewed as being based on fear of loss, with each developmental step representing potential loss.

> Fear of loss means that a mother has to contend with the cultural expectations of maternal power, cultural curtailment of maternal power, has own desire for potency, her conviction of powerlessness, her loving concern to protect her child - and her hate (Parker, 1995, p. 210).

The expression of rage in spite of the previous and subsequent desire not to hurt the object is likened to the failure to mourn loss constructively. The loss is viewed as a threat to the good nurturing internal mother object, with guilt about doing harm to the other. However, instead of guilt leading to mourning, and in the case of the mother dealing with her failure to protect, the results are defenses such as omnipotence, splitting and denial leading to the expression of hostility and the reversal of nurturance.

There is also the issue of how mothers deal with the projections of their children. For example, Chasseguet-Smirgel (1981) has discussed the projected images of the good and bad omnipotent mother, so that the mother is the recipient of omnipotent expectations. For some mothers , such expectations are overwhelming, with the mothers feeling tyrannized and helpless. Added to this are that society tends to view mothers, particularly those who are single parents, as likely to be ineffective, and such mothers are frequently at an economic disadvantage, yet child-care responsibilities are definite maternal social expectations. A maternal ideal is in place that is improbable to impossible to achieve, and its internalization leaves mothers open to guilt and depression as they realize how easy, and threatening it is to display "bad mothering." The narcissism of the mother is in a continual struggle with contradictory and selective demands from the child, from the society, and from herself.

Another vexing issue is the furthering of the gender identity of the child. There is a high probability of significant identification with many aspects of the mother by children of both genders. Part of the parenting process is to make use of the child's identification with the mother, along with the mother's identification with her child, to aid in the establishment of the child's identity. Differential identifications along gender lines are expected, and both a conscious and unconscious continuity between mother and daughter, with difficulties regarding disidentification between mother and son, have been noted (Chodorow, 1989; Herman, 1989). However, Parker (1995) suggests that the obvious similarities of mothers and daughters are exaggerated as an identificatory force, that the relationships of the mother to her own mother and father and to other significant women and men is a more powerful determinant of the degree and type of identifications. Also, Walkerdine and Urwin (1985) contend that the external world repeatedly attracts the mother's attention away from her daughter, or son for that matter, and Samuels (1993) has indicated that it is not possible to accurately predict the results of single parenting, which usually refers to the mother. Further complicating the picture is evidence of mother-daughter sexual interest that can be as powerful as the traditionally posited mother-son eroticism (Welldon, 1988). Maternal desire may be acted upon in disruptive ways, or it can serve to facilitate differentiation through recognition of the other as an object and subject.

The theme that runs through all these accounts of mothering is the significance of the mother for child rearing and the development of the family. The specifics of the impact of mothering, however, are less clear, There is a mother-child interaction, for example, in which both parties play a role, so that mother-blaming in which the mother is viewed as the sole causal agent, or even the main one, is inaccurate as a universal conception. At the same time, the mother is usually the central parental figure for a child while the father is more likely to be viewed as the "other" to the mother. The specifics of being central however, vary for the child. They reflect personal choice within reality and social contexts. The girl's role as a mother will then develop as a fit between what is needed in an actual parental relationship and the fantasy of being a mother, and this fit customarily requires an integration that is flexible and adaptive. The good mother then is represented by taking care of a child in such a way that mutual recognition of subjectivities is continually considered. In contemporary parenting, the healthy narcissism of the mother is expressed in functions that are both traditional (nurturing) and not so traditional (protecting), and are a product of the needs of the family as a system, as well as the dyadic relationship of mother to child, mother to father, and child to father. There dyads include the perspective of each person as both subject and object.

The mutuality of the parents contributes to establishing the specifics of mothering over time. Generally the mother will appear as a significant figure to the child earlier in the developmental sequence than the father, and the roles of each parent will be gendered in many ways. At the same time, the mother can be willing to be a significant "other" at all developmental stages, so that she is not locked into a gender role. This possibility is also open to single parents, or gay and lesbian couples. The parenting role can span gender for identification, recognition, and complementing purposes.

This healthy narcissism can break down in a number of ways that are basically a result of the mother needing to be attentive to personal needs in a way that is detrimental to the child. Examples of such breakdowns appear in failures to resolve ambivalence that restrict the rapprochement of love and hate while creating distorted mother-child adaptations. Another way to view this is an inability by the mother to balance connection and separation for herself and for her child. It is suggested then that any developmental deficits or conflicts that contribute to the skewing of the mother's personal perspective in a way that avoids mutuality, intersubjectivity, and the acknowledgement of ambivalence, represent pathological narcissism that will most likely be translated into pathological mothering.

Thus if there are developmental arrests or distortions in drive expression, this may facilitate seductive or hostile mothering. Inappropriate ego functioning may contribute to various styles of defensive mothering. Difficulties in separation-individuation or even in the establishment of security operations can result in a repetition between the mother and the child. Self-fragmentation makes both the identificatory process and the integration of ambivalence open to one-sided solutions that can undermine the self-cohesion of the child. Regardless of the main motivational emphasis for the mother's expressions of narcissism, there is a high probability of mothers repeating unresolved issues with their children.

The cultural assumption of universal maternal desire that is very frequently incorporated by parents and their children has led to a neglect of the appreciation of ambivalence in mothers, whereas fathers are often expected to be more distant and distinctive parents. However, Greenberg (1991) has emphasized the frequency and inevitability of conflict in all human experience. Internal conflict about wanting to parent is by no means limited to fathers as Parker (1995) has well illustrated in her descriptions of maternal ambivalence. Thus it is useful to view mothering as a narcissistic task where desire for the experience requires a flexible personal perspective that is not necessarily "natural" for mothers. The specifics of good mothering, as with good fathering, are going to vary and are going to have an interactive context. They will include traditional and not-so-traditional activities, and the resolution of ambivalence by making use of what Parker terms its "creative" possibilities. The key element is to have narcissism that fosters an adaptive, mutually interactive family system, where in the case of women, family refers to at least mother and child. This can be facilitated through favorable selective identification, social learning, and evolutionary psychology, but it is finally a matter of personal choice. Thus the healthy narcissism of the mother is reflected in desire and recognition, flexibility and understanding, and separation and connection.

Concluding Comments

The desire for mothering on the part of women is certainly a social expectation and part of her biological and genetic potential. The review by Archer (1996) of evolutionary and social role explanations of sex differences in social behavior lends some support to the existence of a "mothering instinct," but this should not be interpreted as meaning mothers lack mixed feeling about such a role. Thus Parker (1995) illustrates that women are ambivalent about all aspects of being a mother, and Finzi (1996) distinguishes between the desire to produce a baby and the desire for mothering.

Identification with the mother and with femininity certainly play major roles in the desire for mothering, whereas the idea of gaining a lost penis by having a baby appears as a less significant fantasy. In fact it is clear that female sexuality has its own developmental pattern that parallels male sexual development rather than being developed from it or in reaction to perceived anatomical differences. There is an early sense of feminine identity which is brought about by social designation, body awareness, and identifications. This is subjectively perceived and shaped, but it frequently includes an interest in being a mother. The awareness of anatomical differences and the strong libidinal and aggressive desires of the oedipal period are further steps in a process of differentiation that forges an individual identity as a woman.

Finzi notes the continual presence of a creativity in all aspects of maternity which in turn has broader implications, namely "the capacity to give and preserve life can be translated into a particular existential quality that is syntonic with the feminine identity and its specific modality of being in the world and living in relation with others" (1996, p. 4).

She avoids equating actual motherhood with femininity, and thereby excluding non-mothers, by emphasizing the "maternal disposition," but the implication remains of motherhood being akin to the female self. Jordan et al. (1997) indicate that females are raised in a way that fosters relationships and therefore would have a considerable amount of maternal desire. The place of sexual desire in the lives of women is less clearly articulated. Such desire is usually distinguished from male libido, but is not necessarily equated with the choice of a sexual partner, male or female, because this is viewed as many times coming about because of identification with a maternal or nurturing role that involves connection to another person. Also, although mothers do have incestuous desires, the social view of mothers tends to de-emphasize their sexuality, and such a view is often introjected by mothers. Given that this view has been accompanied by women being the objects of desire more often than the agents of desire, there is considerable confusion, conflict, and guilt for women in developing a personal perspective that would emphasize their sexual desire. At the same time it is apparent that women can be agents of sexual desire, can have active, ongoing sexual fantasies, and can desire healthy narcissistic pleasure from intense sexual desire and its expression. The complementary nature of parenting is clear, but the specifics are not fixed, so that mothers have a full range of role possibilities, now even displayed more often in the larger number of single parents who are both mothers and primary caretakers. Healthy narcissism is best expressed in mothering by making use of potentials, but pathological narcissism is more likely to appear in the gendered traditional role as the mother. At the same time, it is understood that traditional roles have their appeal for both genders, but the use of these roles as a pleasurable experience is selective. Healthy narcissism emphasizes the flexibility of the roles without disregarding existing sex-role differences or the need to create an awareness in children of social expectations. Along with that awareness is still another, namely the possibilities for altering repressive social constructions. Gendered dualities, such as communal and agentic, can be unlinked from gender and dichotomization, and experienced in complementary coexistence.

The feminine self within the mother is often depicted as a constellation of "soft" qualities that are in context to the "hard" qualities of the father, but the structures of femininity and masculinity are too complex to categorize without keeping personal perspectives in view. The mother who has been shaped by her environment from birth is always putting her personal stamp on what she is becoming. With greater recognition of the decentering of identifications it becomes apparent that selective identifications continually occur. The apparent movement of a girl to be more like her mother than her father, for example, will be motivated by a variety of personal satisfactions. These include a self-representation of femininity, disaffection for her father, libidinal interest in her mother, fantasied images of motherhood, and these are only some of the possibilities. Staying within the boundaries of that example, which is certainly a frequent possibility, the girl will still both disidentify as well as not identify with aspects of her mother which do not fit the daughter's personal perspective, just as when the girl becomes a mother, she and her child will have selective identifications. The developing female, through conscious and unconscious connections that use learning, fantasy, and relationships, can develop a potential supply of characteristics for her positional identification as a mother. This role is then modified by reality adaptations, but with narcissistic gratifications of love, recognition, competence, strength, agency, and self-integration. Mothering is a developmental step that if taken by a woman provides for additional self development through the development of others. Narcissism is the central feature that can assist or obstruct the adaptation needed to be a successful mother.

V
Narcissism and Psychopathology

The emphasis thus far has been on describing the establishment of the concept of narcissism as both a normal and pathological developmental process. Certain aspects of pathological narcissism have been described, but others need further elaboration. Attention will be given first to the classical manifestations of narcissistic pathology that appear to be the result of child-caretaker interactions. Then an attempt will be made to demonstrate the potential for understanding all forms of psychopathology within the context of distorted personal perspectives that represent pathological narcissism.

Psychodynamics

In the theories of pathological narcissism described up to this point, namely those of Kernberg (1975), Kohut (1971a, 1971b), Bach (1985), Auerbach (1993), and Fiscalini (1993), parental failures are described as the major etiological factor. The specific caretaking limitation varies, however. Thus Kernberg emphasizes oral frustration, Kohut stresses failures to provide adequate mirroring and idealizing experiences, Bach notes a number of difficulties in the mother-child relationship, especially limitations in identification with the symbiotic mother or the separating mother, Auerbach emphasizes maternal anxiety during rapprochement, and Fiscalini suggests three patterns of parent-child interaction that are likely to promote pathological narcissism in the child. These patterns include continual disapproval, unrealistic approval, and approval based on parent-enhancing behavior by the child.

These authors differ in what could be considered the phase of fixation, as oral-symbiotic relative to later stages, although all agree on the force of preoedipal patterns. Constitutional involvement has also been suggested, as for example Kernberg's possibility of a predisposition to excessive anger. In this vein, McWilliams (1994) raises the possibility of increased innate sensitivity to unverbalized affective signals which in turn may be exploited by the child's family. She also suggests that parents of narcissistic patients use their children to fulfill the needs of the parents in an exaggerated way. Typical family atmospheres include excessive criticism as well as inordinate praise. Both atmospheres are evaluative and promote either feelings of never being quite good enough, or uneasiness about the validity of one's successes. Thus the need for a "false self" is suggested as prominent in narcissistic personalities.

The descriptions given thus far of both the psychodynamics and the behavior of people with narcissistic tendencies are broader than what is described as a narcissistic personality disorder by DSM-IV (American Psychiatric Association, 1994). That description is designed to specify symptoms that create a relatively discrete, differentiated diagnostic category. Psychodynamics, common parental patterns, or any other etiology are not suggested. There is an emphasis on the grandiose features of pathological narcissism, namely a pattern of grandiosity, a need for constant admiration, and a lack of empathy. The self-depreciating characteristics have to be implied from the stated diagnostic criteria; for example, the need for excessive admiration suggests a weak self-image that requires continual support. This "flip side" of grandiosity is also noted in DSM-IV as associated features where mention is made of vulnerability in self-esteem, sensitivity to criticism, social withdrawal, the appearance of humility, and feelings of shame accompanied by self-criticism.

Pathological narcissism, however, does not have to be restricted to the narcissistic personality disorder. In fact, viewing such narcissism as a distorted personal perspective makes it applicable to all disorders and provides an additional or alternative way of viewing all pathology that is useful for detection, prevention, and intervention.

In regard to the causes of pathological narcissism, the family environment and interactive childhood experiences have already been designated as the most likely possibilities. However, it is important to be aware that the idea of viewing current pathology as the sign and result of past developmental problems that implicate significant caretakers requires significant qualification and specificity. Generalized predictions from probable developmental-phase difficulties are open to considerable inaccuracy. For example, Parker (1995) suggests that although the mother's childhood development has an effect on her subsequent mothering, it is not directly predictive, and in particular the recipient of bad mothering will not inevitably repeat such a pattern with her or his children. Fonagy, Moran, and Target (1993) emphasize the greater importance of having a reflective self in regard to childhood experience. McWilliams (1994) notes the failure to significantly correlate the degree of psychopathology with the type of drive organization. She suggests that the various psychoanalytic developmental models are not to be viewed as a total or definitive explanation for psychopathology, but that they do have utility, often in combination, for explaining one or more aspects of the etiology of the pathology.

These comments regarding the etiology and development of psychopathology emphasize the subjective nature of disorders. The concept of a personal perspective is reinforced by Chodorow (1996). She points out that although the past is certainly part of the present, the way in which it becomes part of the present is a subjective construction. The value of developmental theories lies in their potential, namely that they describe patterns that are found in a significant number of people, and the knowledge of these patterns provides therapists and diagnosticians with possibilities for understanding patients. However, both the objectivity and the universality of past experiences as predictors of the present are questionable. Childhood patterns are of particular interest in terms of their contribution to subjective experience.

Given the stated reservations it remains useful to look at the psychodynamic developmental suggestions in regard to narcissism. In addition to the possibilities already considered, Reich (1960) focused on the regulation of self-esteem and suggested that the "normal phenomenon" (p. 45) of narcissism becomes pathological when the balance between object-cathexis and self-cathexis shifts so that there is an insufficient object cathexis, and when there are infantile forms of narcissism that are often present in the imbalance. Infantile narcissism is an inability to distinguish wish from reality that results in magical thinking to deal with reality. This is tied to unrealistic views of the self that reflect discrepancies between the self-representation and the wished-for self concept. There is an unending need for compensatory self-inflation. She suggests this arises because of threats to the intactness of one's body coming about as early and overwhelming trauma. She cites the example of a man who was exposed to early and repeated observations of the primal scene which he experienced as destructive. The feelings of catastrophe and annihilation were reinforced by a severely hypochondriachal mother. Such experiences destroyed feelings of pleasure, security, and power and left feelings of anxiety, helplessness, and rage which would require continuous efforts at restoration. It is not possible to establish reparation through identification because the primary objects are so threatening, so there is a movement away from objects towards an overevaluation of the body, particularly the phallus, with a severe disturbance in object relations as well as embarrassment and anxiety about possible physical illness. Another example given is of an obsessional mother who repeatedly used enemas to facilitate early toilet training and fostered the feeling in her son that she had control over his body and that he could not successfully differentiate from her. This was followed by the dissolution of his parents' marriage when he was about three, thereby also removing his father as a force for security, resulting in a need for magical restitution and an accentuated self-awareness.

Although set within the framework of an economic model of narcissism, Reich's accounts of traumatizing parents resulting in a need to excessively value the self are reflective of the subsequent imbalance of self and object interests that have been noted in more recent depictions of pathological narcissism. In essence the child is threatened by primary caretakers both at times when the child is vulnerable and in ways that overwhelm the child. These trauma are threats to the self that are then reacted to by forced and untenable attempts to elevate the self. Thus the foundation for realistic self-esteem is never established, unrealistic ego ideals serve as a replacement which fuel the need for self-aggrandizement which is often at the expense of others and further limits object relations which are already impaired by the lack of appropriate identifications. Neither parent provides a source for realistic regulation of self-esteem, but instead, through their way of relating to the child, they contribute to a distorted overinvestment in a desired, yet unattainable, self-representation. Reich (1960) also notes that the degree to which a desired fantasy will blur reality and become pathologically narcissistic depends on subjective factors which she conceptualizes in terms of ego strength, such as adequate reality functioning and the availability of sublimations. Ego strength is a product of interactive parent-child functioning as well as resulting from constitutional factors and structural conflicts. As a result parental behavior that induces trauma for children has to be considered as having a range of potential impact that involves considerable individual variability.

Rothstein (1979) has pointed out that there has been a notable emphasis on pre-oedipal mother-child disturbances as causal factors for pathological narcissism. These disturbances reflect a range of maternal responses from detachment and hostility to intrusion and overgratification, as well as mothers who vacillate and use both styles. The unifying factor is the mothers' emphasis on their own needs as opposed to the needs of their children. As a result the child does not feel loved for herself, but for her performance when that is approved by the mother. Separation-individuation brings a greater awareness of being alone. Instead of being able to fluidly connect the concept of self-agency with maternal approval, there is an awareness that approval is given very selectively and anger is directed at apparent failures in performance which often seems to include the child's existence. Thus the child has the difficult task of integrating separateness, restricted approval, and mother's expressions of anger which are experienced as destructive rage. The child feels anxious, relatively unloved, angry, and self-preoccupied with needs to control the object.

Based on the degree of deprivation, the child can essentially lose a sense of self, or feel that the self-as-agent is unlovable and defective, or the child may feel lovable only in response to specific acts that can be considered performances to meet the needs of the mother. The need to control the object can be intense, and accompanied by frightening introjects, can require defensive maneuvers such as externalization and splitting. Thus the narcissistic mother begets intense separation anxiety for the child and the need for the child's illusion of perfection to maintain connection to the object. Narcissistic vulnerability revolves around the need to control the frustrating object.

The stage has been set for subsequent power struggles, with an angry self trying to force a frustrating parent or both parents to provide sufficient narcissistic supplies. The lack of integration found in separation-individuation provides a weak foundation for dealing with oedipal issues, particularly castration anxiety. The introjects that dominate are angry, jealous, and retaliatory, so that the stimulation of libidinal incestuous fantasies or representations of wish gratifications intensify the need for illusions of greatness that signify safety but sacrifice reality. Thus Rothstein (1986) describes a state of pathological narcissism that is a defense against separation anxiety that has been engendered by deviations in maternal responsiveness. It is useful to add that this is an interactive process, and that parental frustrations, even if intense, receive variable reactions from children.

Miller (1979) describes the mother who cathects her child narcissistically as one who may indeed love her child, but not in the manner in which the child needs to be loved. Missing features are constancy, continuity, and a structure for the child to experience personal feelings. Mahler (1968) had described this as a failure in the mother's mirroring function when she is insecure, inconsistent, anxious or rageful. The result is a distorted self concept with a focus on presenting a false self. Pathological narcissism is considered a representation of fixation or an incomplete self that was molded by the parents' excessive narcissistic investments in the child. For example, the mother feels deprived by her mother so she now wants to get from her child what her mother is perceived as not having given her. She tries to get this by excessive control of her child so that she can now have someone primarily, if not completely, at her disposal. The child's needs are unlikely to be met unless the child learns to tailor them to meet the mother's specifications.

As a result of such maternal attitudes the child learns to emphasize only feelings and behaviors that are known to get parental approval. Unacceptable feelings are either hidden or split off and under the control of introjects. Pathological narcissism is expressed through a denial of reality in which the child matures and lives as though the original self-object could still be made available. The forms of such an illusion involve either grandiosity or depression. Grandiosity begins with the hope of getting the real object and then switches to struggle with introjects and is tenuously maintained through illusions of achievement. In contrast, depression represents an ongoing fear of losing the object, which although it seems to force a belief that the object is actually available, is sufficiently fragile to leave the person feeling empty. Such a conception of depression can be integrated with subsequent views that defenses against depression are designed to repair damages that have already happened (Brenner, 1991; Renik, 1990). Mayer (1995) has also described depressive affect as the major motive for defense in the phallic castration complex for women which in turn can be a major contributor to pathological narcissism.

Morrison (1986) suggests that desires for uniqueness in respect to an idealized object, and shame and humiliation about such desires, and the vulnerability the desires create are a basic element of narcissism. Rage against the idealized, frustrating other is accompanied by internal despair, reflecting extremes of entitlement and humiliation. Morrison also points out that a number of different features have been emphasized in describing pathological narcissism, all of which have applicability.

These include traumatic conflicts, structural defects, and defensive functioning. Particular areas that have been highlighted include relational difficulties as the lack of separateness, or of differentiation of the other, and self disturbances, as an unrealistic ideal self, reality distortion, feelings of omnipotence, and a lack of self-unity. Also, narcissism has been described as a defense against aggression, as well as against helplessness. The unifying themes are the presence of pathological narcissism in the parents, particularly the mother, which moves children in the directions of maximizing or minimizing the self in unrealistic ways, including combinations of self-distortions

With the disclaimer of universal psychodynamics, let us revisit the interactions between parents and children that often turn up in the life-narratives of patients who are afflicted with pathological narcissism. There is an appealing logic to the view that experiences build upon each other, and that in the development of any person the earliest years of relatively unformed structures and relations offer large opportunities for making impressions, positive and negative, that are likely to affect subsequent personality formation. For example, there has been an enduring view that excessive gratification or excessive frustration during the oral period results in the formation of a dependent personality, although this view is not well supported by empirical evidence (Bornstein, 1996). Originally such a conception stressed the particular psychosexual level of probable fixation rather than the interaction between the child and the caretakers, However, over time greater interest has developed in the interactions, particularly in terms of the internal mental representations that seem to be developed as part of gratification or deprivation. For example, Blatt and Hermann (1992) have found empirical evidence that early experiences with parents can eventuate in specific expectations regarding subsequent relationships. Bornstein (1996) has found that authoritarianism and overprotectiveness have a significant role in the child's development of a powerless self-representation.

Patterns of parenting essentially involve conflict between the perspectives of parents and their children that are power struggles. The newborn infant has the power of personal demands, and the new parents have the power of their reactions. Healthy narcissism reflects a good fit, and pathological narcissism indicates a bad one. The opportunities for the struggle are begun as parent and child are continually involved in the expression and organization of each other's behavior. The ego ideal of parenting is a type of mutuality in which there is sufficient satisfaction of the triad's personal needs so that each person, mother, father, and child consider their interactions a good fit. In previous chapters the ambivalence of the parents has been delineated, and of course the child arrives with a powerful set of needs and little experience in their regulation. Thus the task for the parents is the negotiation of power sharing, and if that breaks down significantly, then the child's self is likely to be damaged in the direction of pathologically narcissistic states appearing in a variety of symptom clusters. What shapes the narcissism into pathological forms? Answers will focus on psychological processes, with the understanding that these can be interactive with social, constitutional, and biochemical factors that contribute to or accompany the psychopathology. The most frequent contributor is parent-child interactions involving frustration-gratification imbalances originally described by Freud (1905) to explain the concept of fixation. However, prediction from specific patterns remains an elusive goal that appears effective only if the various causal possibilities that have been discovered over time are used as working hypotheses subject to reformulation as each personal narrative unfolds in the course of therapy. This process reveals the centrality of narcissism as a personal perspective that essentially organizes behavior. The applicability of such a conceptualization to the range of psychopathologies - psychoses, neurosis, and character disorders - will be illustrated with schizophrenics, depression, and borderline disorder.

Schizophrenia

The DSM-IV criteria for schizophrenia are that the symptoms must be continuous for at least six months, with at least one month of two or more active-phase symptoms which are delusions, hallucinations, disorganized speech, grossly disorganized or catatonic behavior, and negative symptoms such as flat affect, alogia, and avolition. There are significant social and occupational dysfunctions as well. Characteristic symptoms can be considered as an excess or distortion of normal functions (positive, such as delusions) or degrees of loss of normal functions (negative, such as limited affect). Within the specific symptoms, most common are persecutory and referential delusions, and auditory hallucinations. Subtypes of schizophrenia emphasize delusions and hallucinations (paranoid type), or disorganization (disorganized type), or psychomotor disturbance (catatonic type). Anxiety is not mentioned as a distinguishing symptomatic feature, but Karon and

Teixeira (1995) suggest that schizophrenia represents a variety of severe adjustments to chronic terror. They view all symptoms as either signs of terror or defenses against terror.

Karon and Teixeira (1995) conceptualize conflicts with parents, or deficits in parenting, as major contributors to the creation of schizophrenic terror. Parents of schizophrenics often restrict socialization outside the family, thus limiting their children in terms of both information and identification. Another tendency is communication deviance where communication is generally confusing. Intrusive hostility is another likely happening, and Karon and Widener (1994) describe the presence of pathogenic parenting. This is a tendency to act on personal needs without an awareness that such needs conflict with the needs of children who are dependent on the parents, an example of pathologically narcissistic fathering and mothering.

Fantasy structures formed by the schizophrenic in childhood reflect problems with the parents beginning in infancy and reinforced by ongoing child-parent interactions throughout the developmental stages. The child feels extremely unloved, which is equated with abandonment, creating terror that motivates a life dedicated to defending against what is experienced as a strong probability of desertion due to personal deficiency. Attempts are made to deny any badness in the mother and to change the self, or to seek a better object, but these attempts do not succeed. An oral fixation can be considered appropriate as the origin of the difficulties, and throughout life situations keep happening that in turn cause terror that cannot be aided by defenses unless they are major distortions of reality, namely the schizophrenic symptoms. Catatonic stupor represents a fear of dying, and hallucinations are dream states in consciousness, withdrawal avoids the anxiety of attempting to relate to others, and delusions are transferences to the external world with flat affect signifying a chronic state of overwhelming anxiety.

The symptoms of schizophrenia are in different ways distortions of normal processes. These distortions are symbolic ways of dealing with problems in which the unconscious is revealed without the schizophrenic person being aware of the revelation. This is a similar revealing process to the psychopathology of everyday life, but the content is more primitive and obvious, and the mechanism of revealing much more dramatic and unusual. However, their symptoms appear to the schizophrenic to represent the only solution available.

Of course there is the possibility of disagreement about the specific dynamics as well as the causes, but what is striking is the organization of a personal system designed to cope with a chronically episodic set of terror experiences that defy solution as the schizophrenic symptoms and defenses fail to effect a satisfactory fit with ongoing developmental tasks. Framed in terms of narcissism, the schizophrenic patient wants to reduce, avoid, or eliminate terror, and has organized a life around ways to do this that unfortunately cause terror because they disturb others who react negatively, keeping alive the misattunements that have always existed.

Karon and Widener (1994), in an attempt to do justice to the multiplicity of probable causes for schizophrenia, include disturbing life events that are not a result of parenting as well as bad professional guidance and genetic vulnerability. However, their main contributor can be conceptualized as pathological parental narcissism. They grant that other types of patients also may have had disturbed parenting, but see the parenting of schizophrenics as relatively unique in its noxious style and effects. They note that these occur as the parents attempt to deal with the problems of their childhoods, so the parents are not depicted as agents of destruction but as victims of their own difficulties that are in turn increased by their interactions with their children. They stress the unique, subjective view of the child, namely the child's narcissism, as a key to psychotherapeutic comprehension, but this is understandably tempered by a tendency to have at least some universal guidelines. Thus, they assert that very young children perceive their parents, especially their mothers, as causing everything and being omnipotent. This is certainly a possibility, but not a certainty. As Karon and Widener (1994) also indicate, what actually contributed to the formation of schizophrenia in the child is unknown. Considerable research and clinical experience supports the presence of traumatic developmental stages, but universals as to the pathogenesis are lacking. Frequent patterns are signposts, but the construction of a personal narrative remains paramount. It is necessary to unravel how personal constructions were formed that require the reality distortions and personality disorganizations formed in schizophrenia. The more usual types of personal organization are not viewed as satisfying by the schizophrenic and there is a need to alter the personal environment in such a way that it appears as a better fit to the patient. The pathology of the narcissism is that the subjectivity of one individual loses room for the subjectivities of others and in so doing results in a maladaptive self. The parents are in conflict with the needs of the child, and unconsciously satisfy themselves without an awareness of their impact on the child. By so doing they create damage to their self-esteem and become maladaptive in direct opposition to their needs for satisfaction. However, such pathogenesis is also highly variable and emphasizes parental subjectivity. In turn, Karon and Widener note, " Just as schizophrenic patients are also widely different people, so are the parents of schizophrenic patients" (1994, p. 52).

McWilliams (1994) considers schizophrenia as being at the most disturbed end of a schizoid continuum. She indicates that there is evidence for viewing schizoid personalities as temperamentally hyperactive and prone to overstimulation, which often results in a bad fit with caretakers. Oral fixations are suggested, with fears of engulfment and control, and anxiety about fundamental safety. There is a two fold split, between the outside world and the self as well as between desire and the experienced self. Prominent defenses are withdrawal, projection, introjection, idealization, and devaluation. A fear of attachment is notable, as well as a need to maintain personal space as a reaction to a fear of engulfment. McWilliams put less emphasis on anxiety and abandonment fears than Karon, although the presence of anxiety, and the need to develop mechanisms to defend against it, are apparent in both views. Also, both authors acknowledge the probability of multiple or differential etiologies, with McWilliams pointing out that both caretaking deprivation and impingement can be involved. She connects massive anxiety to the possible paranoid component of schizophrenia, where there is a great fear of what others may do to the patient. The paranoia is believed to be engendered frequently by parental environments that were filled with criticism and humiliation of the patient, or family situations in which gross confusion was generated by excessive anxiety of one or more of the primary caregivers. Feelings of emotional isolation are central, and there is a struggle between a very negative self and an omnipotent self. There is often a mixture of confusion about sexual identity and preoccupations with homosexuality. This is in accord with Karon (1989a) noting that schizophrenic delusions can partially be explained in terms of defenses against pseudohomosexual anxiety. This anxiety is not considered reflective of erotic desires, but of loneliness and the apparent greater ease of relating to someone of the same sex.

Both Karon and McWilliams acknowledge the difficulties of establishing anything more than a number of possible conflict and/or deficit producing circumstances that appear to contribute to schizophrenia. However, there is a consensus that there is usually a significant degree of disturbance in the families of schizophrenics, and that schizophrenics use relatively extreme measures to try to cope with their experienced environments. Thus the personal perspectives of schizophrenics are unified to the degree that they need a changed world to live in, and they meet this need by creating an inner world that conforms to their needs while sacrificing reality adaptation. Unfortunately, in turn their maladaptation maintains such pressure on their inner selves that their symptoms and behaviors are ineffective sources of satisfaction. Remediation is extremely difficult because the pathological narcissism limits both the abilities and willingness to consider other perspectives despite a state of pain, that even when fluctuating, has unrelenting persistence that often seems inevitable to the person experiencing it.

An understanding of the pathological narcissism of schizophrenics is reflected in treatment approaches. McWilliams (1994) emphasizes the patient's lack of security and sense of apprehension which she feels will require a more supportive approach than would be used with higher functioning patients. The components of the supportive treatment are demonstrating trustworthiness, educating the patient, and interpreting feelings and stresses of life. Such an approach does not rule out the goal of insight leading to change, as well as the analysis of transferences and resistances, but the context is supportive with a reduction in analytic ambiguity and in turn a restriction on the range of transferences as well as the type of interpretations. The patient's pathological narcissism simply does not shift in response to a conventional interpretive approach, and even with modifications, it remains frighteningly easy to elicit continuations or exacerbations of psychotic responses. In that respect there is no "right" technique, only some better possibilities (Karon & Vanden Bos, 1981). What these possibilities are, in turn, depends upon one's experience in listening to schizophrenics. McWilliams (1994) experiences schizophrenics as dubious about the difference between the therapist and other people who indeed are viewed as threatening. As a result she makes a point of learning what the patient fears from others, and then repeatedly acts in ways that would dispel such fears. The need for the creation of a safe environment in the therapy is, however, difficult to accomplish consistently because I have found that schizophrenic patients are not consistently reactive to my attempts at being consistent as a positive, safe object. There is a fluidity of emotional states that is a result of both frequent and inconsistent reinterpretations of my actions that in turn makes it necessary for me to relearn what is happening, and sometimes schizophrenic patients do not give me that opportunity. My sense if their message is, "do not get in a groove, think that you really understand me and therefore know what you are doing, because I will at one time or another show you that you do not."

McWilliams also recommends emotional disclosure based on the idea that schizophrenics are very emotionally attuned and so they benefit from the therapist's willingness to be known. The idea is that if the patient suspects the therapist of having particular feelings, such as boredom or discontent, an exploration of the patient's fantasies with some validation of the feelings is likely to be helpful to the patient. This approach is in accord with what Busch (1996) has described as making effective use of the patient's ego and facilitating the patient's cooperation in treatment. However, I have not found schizophrenics to be so attuned to what I am feeling. As a result I cannot validate their feelings or thoughts about me as a way to defuse their potential for terror, but instead have to get them to reconsider their impressions. The suggestion by Busch emphasizes the rational aspects of the patient's ego. For me the task with schizophrenics begins with locating that rationality in a specific instance, and then finding a way to use it. Because I find schizophrenic patients emotionally attuned to me only part of the time, I shift my focus to the authenticity of my interest in their fantasy. The difference between my reaction and that of McWilliams may well be a function of our ways of presenting ourselves to very disturbed patients. In my case I find the patients' emotional attunements to be much more in line with their subjective states than with mine. It is possible that the patients are concealing their reactions, or having unconscious reactions to my true emotional states, or that I am unaware of the totality of my reactions. However, what I seem to find is that the schizophrenic patient is dominated by a personal world that limits intrusion and inclusion of others. Thus, although I am there, I am not there, and I have to notice my exclusion and see what I can do with it.

What I am describing is a variation of a suggestion by Busch (1995) that rather than put an emphasis on interpretation and dynamics it be placed on engaging the patient at the level of what can be observed by both participants, namely the patient's subjective, and at least momentarily unique, way of seeing things. For example, a patient tells me that he can discern that I am in danger, that he knows this because a light shone from a golden dome and revealed this to him. I thank him for letting me know, but I tell him that because it is common for people to see things in a variety of ways, I do not feel as if I am in danger. I say that I appreciate his concern and that perhaps I could feel this danger if I could see things the same way he does, but so far I have not seen the light shine from the golden dome. He tells me that he knows that, but I am nonetheless in danger, and that he wants to protect me. I thank him and ask him if he can tell me more about the danger I am in.

In this example I am attempting to validate the existence of his way of seeing things, as well as his feelings in regard to me. At the same time I am letting him know that I do not perceive or feel the way he does at that time. He seems to accept this, and I am then able to have him explore his fantasies about my danger, and subsequently his protection of me. I have not expressed what I am feeling, which is some confusion and anxiety in regard to his vision, nor does he seem sensitive to it. My response is authentic, but partial, and I believe, adequate for the task. My feeling is that telling him more of what I felt would increase his anxiety, but perhaps not. My confusion is tied to the degree of subjectivity that he manifests so that it is difficult for me to know how best to enter his world, to allay his fears, and to help him be more comfortable with realities because he is also confused.

McWilliams directs attention to the schizophrenic's confusion, and responds by reframing feelings in terms of natural responsiveness. Thus the patient's specific anxiety that is relatively unfounded is transformed into an example of acceptable sensitivity and emotional subtlety, in essence a positive with a reinforcement of defenses. I also get this impression of considerable confusion, but the patient's sensitivity seems more selective and sporadic to me, as well as frequently terrifying to the patient, so my acceptance of the patient's productions tends to be qualified with an emphasis on their subjectivity. This is how the patient feels, how the patient sees things, and I want to understand these feelings and perceptions without taking away their distinctiveness. I understand the value of not stigmatizing the patient that McWilliams is aiming at with her deemphasis of the patient's oddities. At the same time, the patient knows from the reaction of others that oddities do exist, and I want the patient to understand that I am aware of the two worlds, the patient's and the world of others that needs to be coped with in a better fashion than has been the case up to that time. In that vein I can concur with the suggestion by McWilliams of examining what is happening to the patient in terms of possible stressors, such as separation, or misconstruals of events. We are certainly in agreement with the need to listen thoroughly to the schizophrenic patient, and we both hear the patient's intense fears and disorganized rhythm, although then we do some different things.

Karon and Teixeira (1995) take note of the difficulty, but not the impossibility, of forming a therapeutic alliance with schizophrenic patients. They stress that because schizophrenics generally are withdrawn in their relationships it will take a considerable amount of time to create a therapeutic atmosphere that a patient will view as being safe. The schizophrenic patient is likely to approach a therapeutic relationship with fear and anxiety that border on terror. On the one hand, the patient is being informed from an external source that the therapy, represented by the therapist and patient meeting and talking with each other, is designed to be helpful to the patient. This help is often depicted in one or more concrete ways, as to get the patient out of the hospital, or to get the patient working again, or any other reality offering that is considered by society to be good for the patient and in turn desired by the patient. Sometimes these suggested goals are wanted by a patient, and other times they are not. However, it is customary that the schizophrenic patient is getting therapy because the patient believes something can be gained, namely the personal perspective finds some attraction, although the appeal is not necessarily congruent with other people's therapeutic goals.

On the other hand, based on the relational history of most schizophrenics there is a good reason to fear that the therapist will try to take away symptoms that the patient considers essential to survive. There are reasons to fear that the therapist may kill the patient based on the narcissistic perspective that regardless of the pain of the patient's current psychic life, it must remain as is. If the patient had not felt a need to create such a distinctive personal world, then the patient would have been different. That need has remained in place and is accompanied by tremendous anxiety in reaction to the possibility of change. Thus the therapist has to face the daunting task of altering this aspect of the patient's pathological narcissism.

The crucial part of the therapist's task is to get the patient to see the process of psychotherapy as potentially more beneficial than dangerous. The schizophrenic patient is accustomed to moving from one dangerous situation to another in terms of self-perception, so the therapist has to diminish the danger of the therapy just enough so that the patient will participate. The therapist begins by offering protection against danger in terms of a holding, protective environment. By virtue of acceptance and understanding that will be limited, but also greater than the patient's previous relational experiences, a different environment becomes open to the patient. This is an environment which could make the symptoms unnecessary, but the therapist can keep anxiety at a minimum by letting the patient have new experiences of safety and from these experiences develop insight into the lack of a need for such excessive defensive measures. The patient's interest in the new situation of relative safety predominating over danger is assisted by the fact that the symptoms are compromises that also have negative components. The schizophrenic's world is an unhappy one to start with, but the narcissistic perspective is not focused on feeling better through the medium of life's ordinary events and relationships. The emphasis is much more on survival, which in turn is perceived as requiring methods that are viewed by others as maladaptive and irrational. The conflict involved between the world's way and the patient's way, as well as the patient's chaotic inner world of terrifying emotional crosscurrents, provide an impetus to consider other offers, such as the therapeutic experience.

Of course it would be both helpful and personally gratifying for the therapist to receive a large amount of consistent trust from the patient throughout the therapy. However, a partial, tenuous form of trust is sufficient to form enough of an alliance to do some therapeutic work, and it is my experience that is usually the extent of what can be put into place, as well as what tends to be there for the course of therapy. I'll call it "good-enough" trust because it works.

The degree of relating, no less an alliance, that is experienced by the patient is significantly dependent on previous relational experiences that have frequently been filled with anxiety as well as ongoing fantasied relations that in their dramatic way emphasize destruction and absorption by others as well as longings for dependency on better, safer objects who can be merged with as well to escape the torment of being isolated and frightened. Thus offsetting the tendency to pull away and stay way from others, such as the therapist, is a dependency on objects and a concern with relationships that occupies a major portion of a schizophrenic patient's life. Apparent objectlessness is deceptive, because the patient is actually preoccupied with others, but not with their reality or their subjective states. Instead, the schizophrenic patient is involved in ongoing unconscious as well as fantasied relational struggles that include a search for new and better objects, although the form and style of such objects can be both elusive as well as concrete but grandiose and improbable. In this search, nonetheless, lies the probability of forming rapid transferences, and such a transference can appear as a therapeutic alliance. While that has the value of getting therapy started, it can be a deceptive beginning in that it looks more promising than it frequently turns out to be.

In looking for improved and even extraordinary objects, Karon (1992) emphasizes the search for a new mother, but the father could be most sought after, or other family members, depending on the personal history of the patient and the prevailing patterns of relational fantasies. Part-objects and fusion of figures as well as identificatory mergers may also operate in the transference, and its positive characteristics that are contributory to the possibility of a therapeutic alliance can undergo rapid transitions as the patient associates to the negative introjects that can quickly fill up transferential space. When the therapist notes a shift from positive to negative transference then the therapist has to evaluate the degree to which this is becoming a block to therapeutic progress, and interpret the transference if it is reaching the proportions of a significant resistance. Because the schizophrenic patient is living more in a fantasied relational world than a real one, the presence of transference is widespread. In this context, Karon (1992) points out that schizophrenic pathology could be understood in terms of transferential reactions to most life situations. Another way of viewing this is to consider it in terms of untempered and primitive subjectivity that is expressed in a distorted narcissism engendered by severely traumatic relational experiences that live on as extremely dangerous and poorly contained introjects.

The existing transferences are to be utilized beyond the formation of relationships in which there is a dialogue of various sorts that permits a working alliance. Transference becomes a pathway to understanding and processing the internalized relational structure of the patient. As these are revealed, along with the terrifying affect that usually accompanies them , the therapist has the opportunity to supply new and different introjects that illustrates relational patterning that is both better differentiated and better connected. Thus the holding environment that is developed by the therapist, and that will need repeated adjustments to be maintained, demonstrates a different kind of parenting than the pathogenic prototypes of the past and offers a new model for positive relationships. In essence the therapist interacts with the patient in such a way that a relatively safe world is developed within the context of therapy. That in turn offers the possibility that the world outside the therapy could also be safer, more tolerable, and of greater interest to the patient so that it becomes less imperative for the patient to live within himself.

The key to doing this is the utilization of empathy in order to be able to see the world through the patient's eyes. Then, with this awareness and knowledge it is necessary to help the patient be aware of the difficulties involved in operating in accord with the patient's view of the world, namely its dangers and the symptomatic measures used to ostensibly protect the patient against these dangers. It is useful in that regard to explore and provide understanding of how such pathological narcissism came into place. This is then followed by discussion of how more effective personal perspectives can indeed replace existing views that are of limited value both as organizers of a personal internal world and of the outer world of consensual reality.

Karon (Karon & Teixeira, 1995) emphasizes the idea that schizophrenic patients can profit from insight in many ways, such as learning to reduce their terror, to accept affects and understand their causes, to see meaning in their symptoms, and to connect symptoms with preceding traumatic experiences. The value of insight is also noted by McWilliams (1994), although her focus is primarily on the provision of a supportive context that highlights the development of the therapist as a safe object, reeducating the patient, and interpreting the stresses of life. I certainly agree with the potential of insight, but I want to emphasize the intermittent accessibility of schizophrenic patients. The alliance fluctuates, the transferences shift, and there are many phases of confusion and misunderstanding on the part of therapists. The patients appear illogical and irrational because they are not operating in accord with a logic that is familiar to most therapists. Also, even when it is well comprehended by a therapist and the therapist attempts interpretations, what ought to be a good fit in its explanatory power may just not make it because the timing is even harder to get right than the context of the interpretation. The schizophrenic world is not designed to let others in, so misconstruals by the patient of what the therapist is literally saying, as well as of the therapist's meaning, intent, and affect, are all likely possibilities.

Karon and Teixeira (1995) point out the symbolic attempts at problem solving and the breakthroughs of what appears as material from the unconscious yet are accompanied by a lack of awareness and a fear of the contents of the unconscious. Such a fear reinforces the need to avoid anyone, such as a therapist, who indeed makes a schizophrenic patient more aware of what the patient is defending against, even if some of that material has been revealed unwittingly. In fact, in reviewing the treatment suggestions made by both McWilliams and Karon and Teixeira, I am struck by the resistances of the patients that require considerable coping efforts by any therapist. This is reflective of the extensive degree of pathological narcissism that is present in schizophrenia.

Karon and Teixeira suggest that in treating schizophrenics the therapist focus interpretations on what is useful to a patient at that time. Of course, the immediate question is, how does one know what that is? There is no definitive answer beyond having flexibility and sensitivity to the patient's variable subjective states, along with acceptance of one's misattunements followed by reparative efforts. The narcissism of the schizophrenic patient is especially difficult for any therapist to sufficiently comprehend because its very quality emphasizes the difference between the patient and the therapist. Although it may well be that anyone could become schizophrenic, a therapist is rarely as pathologically narcissistic as a schizophrenic person, so an empathic reach is repeatedly required and in turn, often restricted. However, if the immediacy of use by the patient can be kept in mind, interpretations are more likely to indeed be useful.

A second suggestion is interpreting from the surface, namely by using reality-oriented explanations first, followed later by more intricate psychodynamic hypotheses. This seems congruent with a suggestion by McWilliams (1995) that interpretation aim at the stresses of life rather than defenses, but seems at odds with another suggestion by McWilliams that a useful technique is interpreting up, namely moving from depth to surface and thereby providing tentative psychodynamic explanations rather quickly in the course of therapy. This possibility is offered as part of an educative approach in psychoanalytic therapy, so it may well be a variation on the need for flexibility in interpretive approaches rather than an example of contradictory procedures. The significant presence of subjective styles in working with schizophrenics has already been noted, and can be seen as a reflection of different personal perspectives. Thus, depending on one's perception of what indeed will be effective with a particular schizophrenic patient at a given moment in time, one may indeed interpret up, or interpret down. Suggested techniques have to be viewed as qualified guidelines. Karon and Teixeira comment, "Whether to interpret early or late, deep or shallow, defense or impulse, is always a clinical judgement that may be in error and may require constant revision" (1995, p. 108).

The work of McWilliams and of Karon and his associates has been presented as outstanding examples of therapists who have been able to work with the extremes of pathological narcissism using psychoanalytic theories and techniques. McWilliams offers a broad-based psychodynamic understanding of psychopathology where the treatment approach to schizophrenics appears to be what could be called supportive-interpretive, with limited use of expressive techniques. Karon appears to consider schizophrenia as a relational and structural disorder which will be responsive to expressive, interpretive techniques provided the therapeutic environment is sufficiently supportive, which is emphasized primarily in the earlier stages of treatment. Although neither of these authors frames the patients in terms of the patients' narcissism, their discussion of both theory and technique supports the presence of unusual, chaotic, and terror-filled subjective states on the part of schizophrenic patients. My own experience with such patients has also given me a similar impression. I believe it is useful, regardless of a particular dynamic theory or method, to actively keep in mind the degree of personal disorganization that is involved for the patients, and the difficulties involved in both finding ways to have it sufficiently revealed and then discovering how to make sense out of it for the therapist, all before it is returned to the patient in some useful form. These patients are operating from personal perspectives that make some type of sense to them, but result in adaptive failures. The point of therapy is to change these maladaptive personal perspectives so that other ways can be seen, attempted, and maintained. Karon and Vanden Bos (1981) have demonstrated that this can happen without medication, that the thought disorder can be reduced, along with the duration of hospitalization, and that further hospitalizations can be avoided. Furthermore, these patients were not the traditional "good" analytic patients, but were minorities with low socioeconomic status. Furthermore, Karon (1989b) has shown from a review of empirical studies that a number of psychosocial treatments tend to be more helpful than only medication. Such results can be viewed as supporting the utility of understanding pathological narcissism as an organizing concept and through the development of holding environments, then being able to make sense out of what looked like nonsense.

Depression

Depression is a characteristic state of mood disorders, which include major depressive disorder, dysthymia, and depressive disorder not otherwise specified. Depression may also be present in adjustment disorders and in bipolar disorders, as well as being substance induced or a reaction to a general medical disorder. Depression as an affective state is frequently part of daily living and a reactive state in terms of disturbing personal and environmental events. Depression is generally described by the patient as feeling depressed, sad, down, discouraged, and/or hopeless and helpless. Sometimes somatic complaints are emphasized as well as persistent anger. The customary presenting picture includes crying, being irritable, brooding, obscuring, anxiety, phobias, worries about physical health and complaints of physical pain. The depressed person makes it clear that he or she is in a negative state that is serious. Guilt, indecisiveness, and negative feelings about the self are pronounced along with a lack of interest in others and an inability to enjoy and derive pleasure from life. As the schizophrenic has created a private world, so does the depressive, but the latter makes others aware of this world of misery, and it is a state that is much easier to understand than schizophrenia.

The "normality" of depression has positive and negative aspects. The positive lie in the fact that it is an understandable state for an observer or listener, thus facilitating empathy and intersubjectivity. The negative lie in the difficulties in distinguishing normal emotional states from disturbed ones, because clinical depression is essentially an increase in unhappiness that at some point crosses a line and is categorized as excessive distress. Thus the pathology of the affective state is based on judgements of intensity, duration, and interference with functioning. Klerman, Weissman, Rounseville, and Chevron (1984) categorize the symptoms of depression as affective, behavioral, attitudes about the self and the environment, cognitive impairment, and physiological alterations and bodily complaints. The affective category includes depression, guilt, anxiety, and different forms of hostility. The behavioral signs are agitation, facial expressions that indicate "looking depressed", psychomotor retardation and slowed speech as well as thought, and crying. Attitudes are self-reproach, low self-esteem, feelings of pessimism, helplessness, and lack of hope, and thoughts of death and suicide attempts. The cognitive impairments refer to decreases in the ability to think or to concentrate. Physiological concerns are the inability to experience pleasure, loss of appetite, loss of energy, decreased sexual interest, sleep disturbance, and bodily complaints.

Thus there seems to be considerable agreement as to the manifestations of depression, although McWilliams (1994) notes that the phenomenology of depression has been restricted by the emphasis on affective aspects that is apparent in putting depressive conditions in the category of mood disorders. She takes particular note of intense sadness, anhedonia, lack of energy, and the feeling that a part of the self has been lost or damaged.

Klerman et al. (1984) point out that all the symptoms do not usually occur in one patient, but there tend to be clusters of emphasis, which is reflected in DSM-IV as well as in descriptions by an individual depressed patient. These authors view depression as having a multiple etiology that could include genetics, childhood experiences, environmental stress, and personality structure operating to a different extent in individual patients. They emphasize interpersonal relations in their treatment approach, and in that sense make it an interpersonal disorder, but they do not consider it as always or solely being caused by disturbed relations. Instead, they base their work on the view that "interpersonal difficulties are usually associated with clinical depression" (p. 51).

McWilliams (1994) notes the possibility of genetic vulnerability to depression, although she indicates the difficulty in separating genetic factors from the degree that depressed parents may pass along their style to their children. She also points out the psychodynamic possibilities of experiencing premature loss, aggression turned against the self, and guilt. Introjection is a major defense, in which where there has been an experience of loss it is coped with by idealizing the lost object and internalizing the negative qualities of the lost object. The depressed person takes the blame for the loss of the object, sees the self as thoroughly bad, and feels pressured to prevent the bad self from causing other losses. This is an approach that fits with turning anger inward rather than at the lost object. It is motivated by a feeling of being incomplete without the object, as though the object had indeed been an essential part of the self. The self is restored by taking in the object, but that includes a sense of badness that results from frustrating experiences with the object. This is combined with turning against the self and idealization. McWilliams describes cycles of admiration for a person, comparative feelings of inferiority, seeking a different object to compensate, and continually failing to avoid loss through the repetition of reactions.

Depression has been suggested as originating from a number of different developmental levels, and having different primary manifestations along with a depressed mood, such as feelings of inferiority, dependency, helplessness, and guilt. Narcissism has been overtly implicated in terms of a need for narcissistic supplies that are not made available primarily due to the unavailability of the mothering object. Blatt (1974; Blatt, Quinlan & Chevron, 1990) postulates an anaclitic and an introjective depression. The anaclitic depression involves feelings of weakness, helplessness, depletion, and being unloved. There are strong desires to be nourished and protected that are connected to an early disturbance in the relationship with the primary caretaker. This disruption tends to occur early in the separation-individuation process with failures in basic caretaking that could be considered oral deprivation. In object relations the focus is on the provision of narcissistic need gratification being tied to the object, thus setting up a fear of loss as well as a reluctance to express anger because hostility could result in abandonment. An oral fixation could be construed primarily in terms of frustration, and based on the actual availability of the object rather than internalization. McWilliams (1984) considers this constellation of pathology to represent a depressive type of narcissistic disorder because of the lack of internalization. Blatt et al. (1990) consider anaclitic depression the most primitive form where loss is coped with by denial and continual pursuit of substitute objects. The emphasis is on the loss aspect of gratification, but this does not imply a representation of what is lost, although it could be viewed as a representation of what is needed but infrequently or inconsistently given, or even that excessive gratification is provided but somehow is coupled with the creation of a fear that the gratification will be lost. The specifics of the etiology of the child's development of essentially an insatiable incorporative mode of relating and accompanying affects of sadness and helplessness as well as continual frustration with objects have not been made clear. They would seem to be a function of the quality of caretaking coupled with possible constitutional vulnerability to the vicissitudes of differentiation that become more apparent in the different stages of separation-individuation. The pathological narcissism is apparent in the feeling of having lost a part of the self in self-object differentiation, or in real or imagined deprivation by the object, as well as an inability to conceptualize self-integration and object constancy or permanence because of the persistent feeling of the elusiveness of objects that are thought to be needed to make the self cohesive. In essence the self is a permanent open wound that defies all attempts at self healing, including finding sufficient gratification in object relations.

Introjective depression is thought to originate at a higher developmental level, apparently phallic-oedipal because it emphasizes the severity of the superego. Primary feelings are guilt, inferiority, and lack of self-esteem as well as reparative desires. Introjection is being used to internalize the "bad" qualities of the caretakers and to blame the self for any apparent deprivations. The ego-ideal is unreachable, the superego is critical, and there are feelings of helplessness and futility in attempting to achieve projected demands for perfection. The object is sought for approval, but even overachievement fails to bring satisfaction because of a lack of belief in approval as a consistent, enduring possibility. There is confusion about relationships, including identity, with considerable ambivalence towards the self and others as well as an inability to resolve contradictory affects. Where anaclitic depression is thought to be engendered primarily by early parental neglect, or the perception of abandonment by primary caretakers, introjective depression is viewed as being engendered by ambivalent parenting that includes significant hostility towards the child. There is insufficient warmth in the parent-child relationship to foster adequate self-representations in the child. This deficiency becomes particularly apparent in the oedipal struggle for affection and positive identifications. Introjection and identification with the aggressor are the major defenses as contrasted with denial for anaclitic depression. There is an attempt to hold the love of the ambivalent object through introjection, which is transformed in a struggle with an ambivalent self now that the object is such a part of the self. Object-representations and self-representations tend to focus on the negative aspects of object relationships because the positive aspects have apparently been insufficient to affect frustration. The positive relational qualities are also so fragile that internalizations reflect a fear of directly attacking the objects or even being that demanding, so the result is uncertainty, guilt, and negative self-judgements, but a continuation of contact with objects. The etiological distinctions between the two types of depression seem to lie in the style of parent-child interactions, because there is the constant of frustration by the caretakers. It is difficult to know why that frustration has a significance for a particular person at a particular developmental phase, but it appears helpful to try to understand ways in which the developmental history could foster vulnerabilities to depression.

For example, Fenichel (1945) considered the loss of self-esteem to be a major concern in depression but distinguished between feelings of abandonment caused by object deprivation and frustration, where the object is desired for caretaking rather than for relational contact, and feelings of disappointment and guilt based on failures in the phallic stage where the object is desired as a source of approval. A similar distinction was advanced by Bibring (1953) who emphasized helplessness as a primary factor in depression, but saw helplessness as being developed potentially from any of the developmental stages, oral, anal, or phallic, depending on the nature and quality of the child's reactions. These approaches do not emphasize interaction, instead seeing the child's experience as a rather direct and relatively inevitable consequence of environmental events. Thus the concepts of fixation and subsequent regressions were considered the best dynamic explanations. In taking that approach it is more difficult to explain the child's states of vulnerability to the caretakers' frustrating and gratifying ways. When the child is viewed as interactive with the parents, then subsequent reactions become more comprehensible. The child is organizing experience from birth in terms of what Morgan describes as "self-definition (e.g., agency, coherence, affectivity, and intersubjectivity)" (1997, p. 319), which could be considered as narcissism, namely a personal perspective. Morgan concludes that the way self-organization continues is sufficiently flexible that the ideas of instinctual fixations and regressions are not applicable. However, fixation could remain useful as a way to understand the degree of temporal impact of interpersonal interactions. The developmental history provides opportunities for understanding the attraction of various repetitive strategies, which can be viewed as regression to fixations, now defined as influential relational patterns of the past. The fixations do not have to be viewed in terms of drive gratification or frustration, although an interactive model of relational differentiation does not eliminate a pleasure principle connected to the satisfaction of wishes. Fixations are instead broadened to include the total perspective of the person regarding past attempts at adaptation that become attractive again as the response to present life events. The attractiveness may still be viewed in terms of a need to reexperience gratification that represents safety and pleasure that is now either missing or at risk, or a need to overcome frustration that is being reactivated by present events and is experienced as an unmet need. The tendency to repeat relational patterns in the hope of at some point "getting it right" exemplifies one such type of frustration. In essence then fixation is freed from an exclusive structural base and represents points and phases of experience.

Also, differentiation based on developmental levels where anaclitic depression is based on an early awareness of deprivation implies the initial experiencing of gratification that is then lost, or inconsistent gratification that poses the threat of loss, or at least some type of early deprivation that is not sufficiently balanced by gratification. Such conceptualizing makes it necessary to utilize an hypothesized merger of symbiotic union that is experienced as more pleasurable than subsequent differentiation. However, this limits the apparent interest on the child's part in differentiation from birth. Thus the idea of a personal, subjective organization of affective states that are part of an interactive process that also includes drive expression would seem to be a more comprehensive explanation for the development of a particular life style, in this case depression.

Blatt (1974; Blatt et al., 1990) describes a model of the development of object representation that does involve increasing degrees of differentiation, but begins with a preoedipal stage which is not congruent with recent findings on infant development (Morgan, 1997). The model proposed by Blatt appears to be primarily within the framework of developing ego structures that consolidate and build upon each other progressively from less to more complexity. Libidinal experiences are considered interactive with levels of representations, although the focus is on the latter. Disruptions in representational development do seem to be construed as fixations in the sense of preventing necessary aspects of future representational development, and those limitations are then represented in the type of depression that is manifested, anaclitic or introjective.

The first level of object representation is sensorimotor where the object is primarily part of need gratification sequences. There is contact with the object in terms of a number of sensory and primitive perceptual modalities, but the object is relatively undifferentiated. This is somewhat more than using the object to provide physical gratification, meaning that there is affectional sustenance as well, but all needs, including object needs, are relatively contextual and interrelated. Actually, the starting point for the sensorimotor stage could be refined to allow for more early differentiation. This would of course change the degree of differentiation at its suggested origin, but it would not alter the concept of increasing differentiation and articulation of both self and object representations.

The sensorimotor stage is followed by perceptual object representation where self-representation and object-representations are clarified but there is a limit in the ability to separate the different aspects of a perception. For example, in contrast to the previous stage where parents would be defined in terms of the provision of gratification or frustration, now the parents achieve a degree of separation, but in terms of global physical characteristics.

This level is followed by iconic object representation based on concrete indicators rather than abstract symbols. An external iconic level stresses functional attributes and an internal level adds dimensions other than actions, such as values and affects of the parents. However, the descriptions do not include complexity. Finally, there is the level of conceptual representation which occurs in the later stages of separation-individuation and with the oedipal resolution, and object representations now should integrate the prior levels. Objects can then be experienced in complex yet integrated ways. Identification and empathy are considered significant achievements of conceptual representation. Blatt et al. (1990) then connect difficulties in developing particular levels of object representations to a vulnerability to a type of depression, which in turn is derived from the type of object relations that are experienced, particularly the emotional quality of the mother-child relationship. Although by virtue of being dyadic this view includes interaction, the emphasis is on object-representations rather than self-representation, or on representational reciprocity.

The level of object representation that is reached includes differentiation, ego structuralization, and the quality of object cathexes. Anaclitic depression appears to be a fixation at the sensorimotor level where there is a strong need to maintain sensory contact with the need-gratifying object. There is anxiety about the loss of the object as the actual and potential supplier of gratification, as well as the use of denial regarding loss as well as object representation so that any apparent loss is diminished by substitution. The self is defined primarily in terms of the quality of significant relationships, namely is there sufficient provision of basic narcissistic supplies.

Introjective depression implies a higher-order fixation, primarily perceptual and iconic representations which are fragmented and ambivalent. Now the fear of object loss emphasizes the withdrawal of love and acceptance, which is defended against by trying to be perfect as well as by guilt and critical evaluations of a self which is considered to be defective. Blatt et al. (1990) have identified both introjective and anaclitic depression in nonclinical and clinical subjects based on subjective experience where self-criticism was the major factor in introjective depression and dependency was the major factor in anaclitic depression. In addition, the severe forms of clinical depression appear to involve a combination of dependency and self-criticism. Thus it appears that a pervasive type of object loss can occur based on familial interactions that threaten the dependency of the child multi-dimensionally so that object-representation emphasizes the holding back of narcissistic supplies by deprivation and criticism. These latter feelings call into question the function of levels of fixation, because the introjective depression supposedly represents a higher order of functioning, yet the severity of depression increases when lower and higher levels are implicated. This raises the question of how the lower level fixation is overcome to the point that the developmental issues of the higher level become activated.

For example, objects at the sensorimotor level are thought to be viewed primarily in terms of their actions toward the child, whereas at the higher iconic level the focus is on the attributes of the parents. These are difficult perceptions to separate, and they are relative, but assuming the presence of such perceptions, they may be more reflective of current experience than past development. In essence, the type of affective experience reported as primary reflects subjective organization that is not necessarily limited by levels of structural representation. Of course the developing person can only act on the capacities available, but the psychological building-block conception of development does not appear to fit the ultimate results, which represent forms of flexible motivational and behavioral organization. Thus Morgan describes a "coloring" (1997, p. 320) of development rather than fixations. However, fixation still seems to be a useful term if it is viewed as a past way of organizing experience that becomes attractive when confronted with present stress. The key issue is the subjective organization of experience, which reflects both capacities and relational interactions in a variety of personal adaptations.

Blatt et al. (1990) describe parental representations depicted by depressives as lacking affection and concern, or being excessively critical. The latter approach could appear under the guise of concern, but is not going to be expressed as affection, so the theme is a failure to meet the needs of the child. The need for gratification and for love tend to become intertwined very quickly, but the subjective reports of patients emphasized differentiated concerns that appear reflective of their previous interpersonal experiences. These findings are useful in illustrating the personal selectivity of affective states. However, the prediction from childhood interactions to present affective symptomatic dominance is notably complicated. As Blatt et al. state, "There can be considerable variation among people in their thresholds for experiencing deprivation and criticism, and these thresholds interact with the actual behavior of the parent" (1990, p. 140).

The results of Blatt et al. (1990) suggest the presence of constellations of depression. These include dependency preoccupations connected to unreliable parents, and guilt preoccupations tied to critical parents, as well as both dependency and guilt that could be related to parents who were both neglectful and critical. However, the type of object representation may not be best expressed as a "level", but as a type of subjective experience. The pathological narcissism of depression is expressed in helplessness and negative feelings about the self and others, and object loss in some form, real, apparent, or imagined is a central feature that is interconnected with the distorted personal perspective so that there is a pervasive sense that a significant part of the self is now missing and is likely to remain that way.

The work of Blatt is of particular interest in suggesting parental patterns that are in turn related to by their children with different types of pathological narcissism. Blatt et al. (1990) note a difference between the characteristic styles of parents of schizophrenics and parents of depressives. The former are described as disorganized and so are their children, who also tend to have difficulty differentiating. The latter tend either to be unresponsive or judgmental. However, the distinction may be more in the interactions between parents and children, because parents of schizophrenics also fit the cold and critical patterns as well, but the terror found in schizophrenics along with their disorganized world is not found in depressives. The subjective appraisal by the child varies in the face of similar parental activities. The specificity of the patterning is further called into question by Bornstein (1996), who refutes the link between orality and dependency that is suggested in the description by Blatt of vulnerability to anaclitic depression, and notes that either overprotectiveness or authoritarianism can eventuate in a pathologically dependent personality, which could also be considered prone to depression. In the work of both Blatt and Bornstein there is an awareness of the importance of structuring the self in response to parenting styles. This in turn can be coupled with viewing parental styles as being structured to react to children. In essence, the interaction between the parents and children has to be viewed as an ongoing process of engagement in which all the parties employ their narcissism. The concern here is with the development of the depressed child, and that is a process of personal organization that from the child's viewpoint is designed to get what is most satisfactory given the type of caretakers and providers that are being made available. Bornstein actually illustrates the elasticity available in making the point that a person with a particular type of personality, and in this case we will use depressed-dependent, can be either assertive or compliant based on the personal perspective as to which behavior is most likely to bring about a desired supportive relationship.

Depression as the result of evaluating an interpersonal situation as in some way overwhelming to the person is a common feature is psychodynamic explanations. Luborsky et al. (1995) suggest that depressive symptoms form because a patient sees an interaction as dangerous in terms of their degree of expected helplessness and concomitant anxiety. In addition to helplessness there is a sense of hopelessness, disappointment and a sense of loss, pessimism and a loss of self-esteem, as well as the possibility of suicide. Anger may also be expressed towards others, although it is more often turned inward, The source of vulnerability to depression, in this case the feeling of being helpless in a psychologically dangerous situation, again appears to be vested in developmental experiences. Mayer (1995) notes a connection between depressed feelings and a concern with what is believed to have been lost.

Depression represents a form of pathological narcissism in which the person approaches life as though it was beyond the individual's abilities to be adaptive. The constant in depression is the feeling of being depressed, with other common feeling states and behaviors that are congruent with these affective states, such as feeling and acting helpless or hopeless or dependent. These feeling states as ways of life appear to be related to family situations in which the child's best survival mechanisms were depressive. Caretakers who foster an environment in which there is the threat of loss that is perceived as lowering the child's self-esteem appear to be major contributors to depression in their children. However, the child-parent interaction is more significant than the parental approach to the child, because the lack of nurturance and criticism that is often found in parents of depressives does not always have that effect on children. Furthermore, certain parents are more likely to respond to frustrating children in ways that could engender depression, whereas other parents handle frustration in far more adaptive and constructive ways.

For depression to develop as a personal perspective the person has to consider that such feelings and behaviors are the most likely to bring about the satisfaction of their needs. Depression appears self-defeating because so much is given up, but for the depressed person there is affective safety that is not considered as available through more active participation in life, and if life is sufficiently burdensome, than complete withdrawal from its pain through suicide, can have a compelling logic. Intended suicide is the consequence of needing to win out over intractable psychic pain. The safety of withdrawal, which is represented in the various aspects of depression, needs to be emotionally countered by the appeal of involvement, and that is very difficult to bring about when depression is severe.

The general psychotherapeutic approach of acceptance, understanding, and empathy certainly appears useful in depression, but it is frequently rejected as insufficient and inauthentic. Logic regarding erroneous beliefs about both the self and others also may fall on deaf ears. These approaches are expected in a sense because the depression is a reaction to other people's interest in getting the patient to behave in some way that is not the patient's choice. Thus therapists who understandably see themselves as offering help and hope are very likely to be distrusted and pushed away, either by a lack of responsiveness or by the patient's anger. In essence the patient is making a statement that he or she cannot or will not do whatever it is the therapist seems to want the patient to do. Freedman (1986) has suggested that depressive patients are particularly unreceptive to both the content and the timing of the offerings of others. Thus the understanding of the patient's narcissism is particularly useful because it is a logic for the patient's behavior, and in turn provides an entry into the patient's world that is not threatening to the patient, provided of course there is not an implication that the depression must be given up. The patient may actually say that he feels awful and desperately wishes to feel better, to which the therapist can agree, but that does not mean the patient wishes to act as an agent to change the feelings or believes that the therapist has some palatable possibilities for change. It is as though the patient wishes to be different without having to change.

However, the personal narrative does contain possibilities because it clarifies the patient's point of view, and the ongoing interaction with the therapist adds to the possibilities because even in withdrawal and in a patient's anger, there appears to be a search for the "right" kind of contact that will allow the pain of depression to be lifted. It is difficult for the therapist to discover this "rightness," and easy to be mistaken. Also, the behavioral manifestations, such as dependency and pessimism, can feel overwhelming to the therapist. Depending on the listener, a certain amount of depression is relatively easy to respond to with empathy, but when that threshold is crossed there are temptations to tune out, to avoid, to confront, and to get personally depressed, all of which have to be processed by the therapist so that the hopelessness does not become destructively contagious.

Of the psychodynamic conceptualizations available, I have found a focus on a lost part of the patient's self to be particularly useful. This often appears in the patient's emphasis on the perceived loss of another, but upon investigation appears more as a feeling of being fragmented, so that the sense of helplessness, as well as anger and guilt, are quite strong. For example, a woman described her lengthy marital relationship to me as a source of great unhappiness because her husband was both distant and demanding. She said she was not angry at him, although he had been unfaithful a number of times. She said it was probably her fault, but that she just was not a very sexual person. She felt as if she had lost him, and at the same time she contemplated divorcing him. It became clear over time that she did not like him, but whenever I tended to be empathetic, she blamed herself. If I shifted and expressed concern for her in terms of her difficulties in feeling for him, she became angry at me and saw me as being a part of a family situation in which she was the least favorite child. When I noticed her anger, she apologized. The process of therapy felt circular to me in that no matter where we started we would both end up as wrong, and I expressed this. Her response was to become more depressed, now commenting that she was probably a "hopeless case." I reassured her that was not the case, and I added that I felt she had been losing parts of herself as she moved through her life. She expressed some interest in understanding what I might mean. I told her I had this image of her family kind of "nibbling away" at her, and that continued in her marriage, and perhaps the therapy felt like that too, sort of well-intentioned efforts to relate to her that kept missing who she was. She told me that she liked to help people, and I said I could feel that, but the people seemed to not really be there, or if they were there, then they left. Her father had died when she was an adolescent, and she made the point that she couldn't help that.

When she had discussed the death of her father previously she had often implied it was in some way her fault, so this was a shift. I asked her if she felt lost after he died, and she said, "sort of." Her reluctance to elaborate was ultimately explained because she had symbolized her father as her "good right arm," and she had for months after his death tried to do most things using her left hand as though the loss had been an actual part of herself. This theme, although not experienced so literally, reappeared in other significant relationships and became a way for us to understand her depression and for her to alleviate it by actively pursuing the "lost" parts of herself.

Borderline Personality Disorder
          This disorder is a particularly messy one with a broad range of pathology included in the DSM-IV category so it is often difficult to attach the label with certainty. Meissner (1988) describes a borderline spectrum, as does Goldstein (1996) and Chessick (1997), the latter describing the spectrum as "a heterogeneous group of patients with a variety of levels and degrees of pathological personality functioning" (p. 445). The DSM-IV description of borderline personality disorders includes patterns of intense and unstable relationships, identity disturbances, impulsivity, self-destructive behavior, affective instability, intense anger, paranoid ideation and dissociative symptoms.

          Kernberg (1984; Kernberg, Selzer, Koenigsberg, Carr, & Appelbaum, 1989) has suggested a conception that is both descriptive and structural, namely the borderline personality organization which emphasizes identity diffusion, defenses, and reality testing. Identity diffusion refers to the absence of integration of self and others, experienced by the patient in ways such as continual emptiness and contradictory perceptions of others. The defenses are primitive, as splitting, primitive idealization and primitive devaluation, projective identification, denial, and omnipotent control. The "borderline" between this disorder and psychosis is crossed in terms of level of defenses, which appear significantly different from the higher order defenses of neurosis, such as repression. Splitting appears as a particularly characteristic defense which is aimed at separating contradictory experiences of the self and others. The other defenses are related to splitting. For example, in projective identification a disturbing impulse is projected onto the object yet continues to be experienced by the subject; the object is feared as being controlled by the impulse; and, there is a need to control the object by trying to stimulate behavior in the other person that would indicate the existence of the projected impulse in the object (Kernberg, et al., 1989).

The "borderline" between neurosis is crossed with the retention of a capacity for reality testing. There are, however, alterations in the subjective experiencing of reality (things feel odd) and the relation to reality (inappropriateness) as well as ego weaknesses, such as poor impulse control, superego weakness, as immature values, and continual relational disturbances. The borderline personality organization depicted in this manner is a broad classification that also includes histrionic, narcissistic, schizoid, paranoid, and antisocial personality disorders (Kernberg, et al., 1989).

In contrast to a typical neurotic personality where the emphasis is on structural conflict in the oedipal situation, borderlines show primarily preoedipal conflicts, although representations of the self and of objects are mixed with oedipal representations. Also, instead of intrapsychic conflicts being primarily repressed, the conflicts appear in dissociated ego states reflecting the operation of splitting. Intrapsychic conflicts are expressed through primitive internalized object relations occurring before structural consolidation. Primitive self representations and primitive object representations are linked by primitive affect. There is a fixation in the rapproachment subphase of separation-individuation based on pathological parent-child relations. The cause of such relations could be constitutional or experiential or some combination, and usually involves a strong aggressive component (Kernberg, et al., 1989).

This theory is a mixture of structural and relational components. For example, the assessment of the borderline patient can be viewed in terms of the strengths and weaknesses of the ego. The treatment focuses on the transferential reactivation of primitive past internalized object relations to significant others. These relations are a mixture of reality and fantasy, and tend to be distorted under the influence of drive derivations linked to chaotic affective states. The relational aspects seem to stress the influence of the parents, particularly the mother, more than the mutual interaction.

The considerable heterogeneity of the borderline personality disorder has always been remarked upon, and still prevails (Goldstein,

1996). Meissner (1984) has suggested a number of common features that can be found within a spectrum of different types of borderlines. These features include primitive relationships, such as intense dependency, that are essentially unrealistic and focused on only part of the other person, so that overall relations are colored by self involvement, demands for object love, and inability to accept object connections when they are made available. The result is such fragile object-constancy that relations to objects are severely impaired by the mixture of intense need and intense fear of the other person. There is a rather constant and disruptive shifting of introjective constellations that results in deficient cohesiveness of the self, in essence an inner instability, and a potential for regression.

Meissner (1984, 1988) suggests a model of borderline personality organization which illustrates factors that can derive from genetic, organic, and dynamic processes. These are potentially converging influences with a developmental process as their core. This process will result in a structure anchored in internalization and eventuating in a personality organization. The basis for pathology lies in fixations and defects reflected in self development. The self is viewed as a superordinate concept including and integrating the other structures of id, ego, and superego, but not reducible to the totality of its parts as equivalent to the person. "The whole, in this case, is to some extent greater than the sum of its parts" (1984, p. 443).

Meissner suggests that introjective organization occurs along two dimensions, narcissistic and aggressive. The narcissistic involves superior or inferior introjects, whereas the aggressive has aggressor and victim introjects, and these are polar dimensions. In severe psychopathology these introjective dimensions dominate the person's sense of self. Thus the narcissistic personality is differentiated from the borderline by being organized around narcissistic elements of introjects, primarily preservation of the self through maintenance of narcissistic supplies. The borderline personality is instead organized around a complex of narcissistic and aggressive issues, including being both victim and aggressor. The dominance of aggressive derivatives is related to a strong degree of parental hostility and rejection so that there is a lack of integration of good/bad images of objects and of the self, splitting, and projected hostility. The narcissistic personality is viewed as having a stronger self-cohesion, although with a vulnerability to object loss.

The psychodynamic explanations of borderline personalities have been numerous and illustrate the difficulty in providing an adequate theoretical formulation for a disorder that is in itself very difficult to define, yet a sense of its presence, of "borderlineness" is often experienced by therapists in reference to certain patients. In this vein, Chessick comments, "a substantial segment of psychotherapeutic practice is made up of...patients who fall more or less under this DSM-IV rubric" (1997, p. 441).

Instinctual forces have been depicted as threatening the ego to the point of excessive dependency or control. Instinctual phase dominance is unclear, with oral and anal fixation predominating, especially pregenital and genital strivings influenced by the aggression. Such aggression is also projected to the parents so that they are viewed as destructive.

Defensive failures are sometimes seen in temporary psychotic regression, with the transient nature separating the borderline from psychosis. The use of splitting as a primary defense rather than repression provides a distinction from neurosis. In addition to the emphasis on the use of primitive defenses, other ego weaknesses have been postulated, as poor impulse control and limited tolerance for anxiety. In some contrast to specific ego defects, developmental deficits have been suggested that are seen as resulting from disturbed parent-child relationships, particularly during separation-individuation. Another possibility is narcissistic entitlement because of a vulnerability arising from maternal withdrawal that threatens the cohesiveness of the self. Defective object-relations are also implicated, as well as identity loss and the creation of a false self.

All of these approaches have limited explanatory power in that one or more seem particularly applicable to certain borderline traits but not to others. Also, the theoretical framework of different aspects of borderline pathology becomes questionable. Thus, although splitting is an often observed phenomenon there is disagreement as to whether it is a defense or a developmental arrest. In addition, it is not found solely in borderlines (Meissner, 1984). Then, even though the rapprochment phase is usually highlighted as the time of original difficulty, splitting may be traced to earlier levels. The idea of being able to predict borderline characteristics from difficulties at specific developmental phases is questionable, a problem that has been noted in regard to all forms of psychopathology. Meissner concludes "...conceptualization of a link between a phasic developmental failure and a specific form of psychopathology cannot be consistently maintained" (1984, p. 53).

A distinction is drawn between the vulnerability of narcissistic personalities and borderline personalities in terms of a greater danger of disintegration and less reliance in borderlines, but it is unclear as to the reasons for this. Regressive self-fragmentation has been noted in both disorders. Meissner's (1984, 1988) suggested distinction between narcissistic and borderline disorders based on the distribution of introjects also seems to run into the problem of overlap. For example the concept of superior-introject in the narcissistic disorder could be equated with the concept of aggressor-introject in the borderline disorder if a distinction is not drawn between narcissism and aggression as separate dimensions for the organization of introjects. Instead, the superior-introject is the aggressor-introject, and the inferior-introject is the victim-introject. This raises the possibility that the borderline disorder represents a particularly severe form of representational distortion. The disturbance is in the constancy of representation, and Auerbach (1993) has suggested that narcissistic personality disorder centers around difficulties in evocative constancy that indeed are similar to what happens in borderlines, but less intense. Thus the distinction between pathological narcissism and borderline pathology is far from clear. The borderline disorder could be viewed as representing a type of pathological narcissism where the personal perspective is dominated by shifts that are particularly intense in their manifestations. Notable among these are aggressive superiority and vulnerable inferiority, defensive breakdowns with impulsivity, and self-fragmentation, all aimed at preserving the self as best as one can in the face of what appears to be overwhelming threats.

The suggested psychodynamics for borderline disorders involve a "stacking effect," namely that disturbances in psychosexual and psychosocial developmental phases tend to accumulate so that multiple fixations appear likely and in turn, multiple regressions. At the same time there are varying degrees of adaptation that limit the probability of a slide into psychosis, and at times make it appear as though a neurotic level of functioning is being approached. Usually the emphasis is on the nearness of the borderline to psychosis, and therefore understanding dynamics in that context, although there is also general agreement about borderline personality structure representing a range or spectrum. For example, in 1968 Grinker, Werble, and Drye had described four subtypes moving in severity from the psychotic border to the neurotic border. The symptoms of the former were inappropriate behavior, reality testing and identity problems, and excessive hostility, whereas the latter involved anxiety, anaclitic depression, and narcissistic features. Gabbard (1990) notes the stable unstability, or the unstable stability of borderline patients. Major psychodynamic models have attempted to provide some key mechanism of distinguishing the borderline organization, but being specific has customarily been met with subsequent criticism. Thus ideas such as distinctive constitutional aggression, inadequate parenting in a particular developmental phase, specific introjects, or cognitive deficits (Adler, 1985), have all been contested. Clearly there are relational difficulties, and Benjamin (1996) has suggested four major developmental features that stress interpersonal issues. These are the prevalence of chaos in the family that is either sought after or created; traumatic abandonment involving abuse and the idea that the abandoned person is bad and so deserves punishment; family norms restricting autonomy, despite leaving the child alone, and encouraging dependency including self-sabotage; and, the family responding with nurturance to depression and illness. There is a theme of inconsistency in which gratification and frustration are inappropriately provided, but this theme is not specific to borderlines. However, as Meissner (1984) has noted, the borderline processes experience in a particular way that could eventuate in distinctive responses, exemplified in the idea that the aggressor-introject and the grandiose-introject represent differential affects as opposed to emphasizing their similarity.

The distinctive processing suggested by Benjamin involves internalizing abandonment and so engaging in impulsive self-destructive behaviors. Feelings of emptiness are related to internalizing neglect and associating it with feelings of boring aloneness and danger. Fear of abandonment is related to trauma and being a bad person, and the family attraction to chaos accounts for the borderline patient's instability. Anger appears as an attempt to block abandonment and get nurturance, and identity diffusion is a reaction to inconsistent parenting as well as a protection from internalized parental abusers, which also is related to paranoid feelings. Dissociation functions as a way to shut out stress, as well as a method to try to handle the contradictory parental standards.

As with other dynamic explanations, this works better as a retrospective explanation than a predictive one because of overlap with other disorders, and because it remains at an explanatory level above the basic question of why the patient internalizes particular concepts and develops particular defenses when other possibilities exist. For example, children react in different ways to the experience of abandonment. Grant the possibility of temperamental differences as well as neurobiological correlates, but in trying to understand the psychological ones, it is crucial to keep in mind the human potential for subjective reactions to trauma. Thus, although Benjamin (1996) believes that incest is a common developmental feature for borderlines, she acknowledges that not all incest victims become borderline. Again, as in other forms of psychopathology already described, there is a personal perspective that represents the individual's view that the symptoms displayed are the necessary solution to existence. Because the solution is actually maladaptive, it is pathological narcissism.

The borderline patient has a reputation for being difficult to work with in psychotherapy. The uniqueness of these patients has been noted by Goldstein (1996). Chessick makes the point in stating, "...our task as therapists with these patients is to be flexible enough to hear what each patient is attempting to tell us about what sort of therapy she can tolerate, ..."(1997, p. 447).

In that vein I want to emphasize two related usual borderline approaches to therapy, namely a shifting and angry style of relating. This female patient began her session by talking about a time when her "feelings were petrified," and asking if the therapist remembered that time because it was very frightening to her and she did not want it to happen again. The therapist remembered a period in which she often described feeling "numb and dumb," but he was not sure this was what she meant. However, he felt that she was asking for his help, and that was more important than clarifying her statement, so he responded by telling her that he would indeed help her not to feel that way again. She seemed to dismiss the concept of help and asked him if he thought she was now starting to feel petrified. He had a number of associations, including that petrified was the absence or opposite of feeling, and that by offering help she had experienced him as being critical, affirming a regression. He felt rejected as he struggled to understand what she wanted from him. He then asked her how she was feeling, and she told him she was afraid, afraid of going back, or of already being there, and that no one could help her, and she concluded by asking why anyone would want to help her anyway.

He noticed that she had removed him from being the potential helper and broadened the issue to "anyone," but that she sounded desperate. He responded to the desperation by noting that she clearly had issues to worry about, and she then agreed. She seemed to feel understood, and she talked for a while about a specific child-rearing concern of hers. While doing that she expressed a fear of inadequacy in case the country was ravaged by a terrible disease. He asked her what disease she might be thinking about and she talked about countries where children were starving. She went into a lot of detail regarding the food supply in various African countries, and then accused him of probably thinking of the Holocaust because she knew he was Jewish and that's all Jews think about when somebody mentions a disaster. He had not been thinking about the Holocaust, but rather that she had a need to get distance from herself and from him, and that she had started toward him and now needed to pick a fight with him to get away. He felt that interpreting the anger directly would cause further anger and not be productive, so he sidestepped it and commented that she was feeling someone closing in on her. She agreed and said it was her mother, who had recently made a negative comment about the way the patient was raising her child. The rest of the session was spent talking about her experiences with her mother and the effects she senses these experiences have had on her. Thus the session went from being unusual and requiring considerable reflection and specialized intervention on the therapist's part to being usual, although with a bit of dread by the therapist that it would again shift and he would not again be able to handle the change effectively.

The countertransferential potential with borderline patients is always very large. The activation of their personal perspectives is variable and unpredictable beyond the probability that the therapist will be attacked. The introjection of the bad object as well as the projection of badness, feeling vulnerable, and needing to protect the self all coexist with dependency, but the picture is frequently chaotic and it is often very difficult to know how the therapist's responsiveness is going to be treated. The patient points to a direction in this example, her critical mother now part of her critical self and projected to the therapist who must also be seen as critical. She puts many obstacles in the therapeutic path. She tries to make their relationship chaotic and untenable, yet she also needs him to help her replace that critical introjected mother who still exists as a critical reality. He has to understand her pathological narcissism as a disturbing mixture of feelings that will often move her away from comfort because distress has always been so important. As Benjamin notes in describing the borderline's philosophy of relating, "My misery is your command" (1996, p. 115). I have tended to experience it a bit differently in the therapy sessions, namely "Your confusion is my command."

Comment

In this chapter, I have tried to make the following points; that psychopathology is primarily an expression of a personal approach to life, that psychodynamics are useful clues to understanding the approach provided the personal narrative is explicated and respected, and, that the concept of pathological narcissism is a useful one, either as an additional framework or as the basic point of reference, for both explaining psychopathology and making interventions.

In regard to the first point, the different symptom patterns can be thought of as the person's attempt to organize life, to relate to the self and others, in a way that is deemed "subjectively best." Often the way is recognized by the person as deficient, but it still is experienced as "best" because it is the only way the person feels he or she can behave. The pathology lies in the maladaptiveness of the behavior, which leads to the second point, explanations for why any patient feels and acts restricted to pathological solutions.

Psychodynamic explanations emphasize various developmental processes which invariably implicate the patient's significant caretakers. Excessive frustration or excessive gratification are the patterns that tend to emerge as related to subsequent pathology. The emphasis may be on drive expression, structure formation, relational interaction, or self expression as major motivations, or these may be combined in some way because motivations overlap to varying degrees. Regardless of the emphasis, it is generally not possible to be specific enough about etiological probabilities, for example parental rejection, to predict the specifics of pathology. However, the unfolding of any personal narrative can provide the specifics of trauma, defense, and adaptation for interventions to take place, and the suggested dynamics for diagnostic categories are potential areas of therapeutic exploration.

Thus we arrive at the third point, the most effective way to look at the patient. The existing psychodynamic possibilities have acknowledged limitations. The concept of narcissism, defined as a personal perspective, is suggested as one way to improve understanding and therapeutic efforts. It emphasizes the subjectivities of all involved and the complex variations of all behavior as well as the relativity of objectivity. Every person is thought of as organizing themselves in a way that is unique, similar to others and capable of relative categorizations, yet essentially distinctive.

VI
The Narcissistic Hour

In a sense, every session, every therapy or supervisory hour, is narcissistic because of the inevitable subjectivity of the participants. The emphasis here is on the narcissism of the therapist or supervisor, which appears first in the preformed manner of approaching the session, the theoretical choice that leans one in the direction of favoring certain emphases. Then there are other subjectivities, such as how the therapist feels, psychologically and physically, during the session, as well as the reactions that are experienced, expressed or not, during the session. The range of mutuality believed in by the therapist will be reflected in the degree of asymmetry presented. However, it is my impression that there is only subjective objectivity, and in turn, because the point of all sessions is supposed to be to help the patient, that all subjectivity ought to have an objective thrust to it. Of course the latter is not always accomplished so that some sessions are more for the therapist's benefit than the patient's, but that is not the goal, even when therapists are apt to be confessional.

This chapter will present, through clinical examples, the workings of therapists' narcissism first in therapy sessions, and then supervisors' narcissism in supervisory sessions. The examples are taken, in disguised form, from the author's experiences and they reflect the theoretical and technical preferences of the author, which tend to be integrative, as well as the relational tilt of contemporary practice. The purpose of these illustrations is to point out the subjectivity involved and how the therapist's narcissism can be profitably put to use as well as to show how it can be a hindrance, particularly where it goes unnoticed, is denied or otherwise used defensively to avoid the patient or collude with the patient. The words "analyst" and "therapist" are used interchangeably in the section on therapy sessions, as are the words "supervisee" and "therapist" in the section on supervisory sessions.

Therapy Sessions

The patient was a candidate in a psychoanalytic institute. He was describing to his analyst how a supervisor in the institute had, during a supervisory session, called the therapist by his patient's name.

The analyst asked, "What did you do?"

Upon reflection, the analyst did not consider this the best question to have asked. She felt it would have been better to have asked him how he felt, but she believed she knew that he did not like being identified as his patient, who the supervisor had disparaged during the session, and he did not like his name being forgotten. At least she knew she would not have liked all that. However, she did not give him the opportunity to tell her what he felt because she wanted him to act. Her desire was partially based on her experiencing him as too passive, and also on her dislike of that particular supervisor who was very confrontational and critical of the therapist's patient. She believed she would have raised the issue with the supervisor had she been the supervisee, and she wanted her patient to be her.

The patient replied, "I didn't say anything."

Now the therapist asked, "How did you feel?"

He said, "I was angry but I was afraid to bring it up."

She said, "Well, you've told me how she often tells you to watch for patients doing things to you that you let pass, and that you need to be more confrontative."

He agreed, "I probably should have said something."

"But you're afraid of her?"

"Yes, she reminds me of my father, always picking at me, I could do nothing right. I just want to get through this supervision, not rock the boat."

The therapist said, "I understand."

She experienced a sense of disappointment nonetheless. It was true that he could "pass through" the supervision, and that he could get a bad evaluation from the supervisor if he challenged her because the therapist knew her well enough to suspect that the challenge would probably be defended against. Still the continued impression of the castrating father disturbed her. At the risk of being overly attached to her need for the patient to be active, she made an interpretation.

She said, "You're afraid you'll kill her."

"It could be," he said. "I know I feel I let my father die, by not doing enough. I could have done more, and I didn't, and I killed him."

Now she felt a certain exhilaration. She had been a bit off target but close. She said, "I think I see. You would like to kill her, and perhaps you can, just by doing nothing."

She thought, perhaps this is the way we all kill our parents, by ultimately not doing anything so that we can save ourselves, because if we do just one more thing, it will be our last thing, and it will still not save them. She thought of all she had done to save her father, yet to no avail, and actually how impressed she had been with the patient's efforts to take care of his father, a tyrant who was very hard to love, in contrast to her father, who was so loving.

The patient said, "I want her to be like my mother, and I did not argue with my mother, but at some point, I suppose, I knew it was time for her to die. I told the supervisor about the death of my mother, that it was recent."

"You want to transform the supervisor, bring your mother back to life?"

"I miss her. I still mourn her."

The therapist felt as though she wanted to touch him. She could feel his sorrow wash over her. She mourned her father, he mourned his mother, and they were alike that day in a way she had never anticipated.

The next session, the patient said to her, "I mentioned to my supervisor that she had called me by my patient's name."

"What did she say?"

"She said, well I've done that in a number of sessions. Why didn't you bring it up before this?"

They both chuckled at the irony of the exchange.

The therapist said, "I guess we cannot raise the dead after all."

He made no comment or inquiry about her use of "we," but there was a tremor in his voice as he resumed talking about his fond recollections of his mother. The therapist reflected on how forcibly she had included herself in her previous comment to the patient. She wondered what that had meant to him, but decided not to ask him, at least, not at that time.

Comment

There are of course many paths not taken in this example and that will be true in all the examples. Our interest here is how the therapist's narcissism was at work. She came into the session focused on the passivity of the patient. He was too passive for her, both on a personal level and then she objectified that to make his passivity a therapeutic problem. At the same time, passivity was a character trait of the patient's that had often caused him to suffer, and his aggression was generally expressed in a passive-aggressive manner. Thus it was easy for her to get beyond her own direct assertive style as the impetus for pursuing her line of inquiry with the patient. Then the incident with the supervisor gave her an opening that fit well with what she saw as a central issue for the patient. Also, she disliked the supervisor's style, which she saw as excessively critical, overly defended, and designed primarily to keep the supervisee confused. Thus, she wanted her patient to attack the supervisor, as she wanted to do herself, and in fact would have done if she was the supervisee.

    She recognized that the supervisor was a transference figure for the patient, but she bypassed that issue and at the time did not think of her own transference toward the supervisor. She was going after a present situation, suspecting before she asked that her patient had not confronted the supervisor. She wanted him to do it so much that it was not until she asked him what he had done that she realized she was ignoring the patient. She could imagine what he felt, what he wanted to do, and added in what he should do as well as an intent to get him to do it.

    However, when she senses her attempted takeover of the patient and begins to explore his feelings, then new directions emerge. The patient is not mainly concerned about his lack of assertiveness with the supervisor, nor is he looking for assertiveness training. He is reliving his disillusionment with his father and in particular he is mourning his mother. The mention of the patient's father triggers a reaction in the therapist, namely associations to her beloved father, and to her much less loved mother, and she uses these associations to interpret his fear of death as well as his guilt about his parents dying, and the other side of the ambivalence, his desire to be free of them, particularly his father.

    She emphasizes fear and hostility first, because they came to her as a first line of defense against the sadness and guilt she has about her own father's death, but she is able to move as the patient moves into mourning. Then, although she does not discuss this directly with the patient, she does overtly bond with him by her use of the word "we," adding an intersubjective dimension to what is happening between them. She also takes note of the relationship between them, his reaction to her, and the, at the moment, unexplored transference, because she had begun the session in an identification with the agressor, the supervisor, because she, the therapist, was also ready to be critical, at least by implication, and in the next session he may well have responded to the implication because he reports taking some action. However, the therapist now has shifted her focus and can better understand the patient so the neither of them spend time on what he ultimately did with the supervisor.

Of course why the patient took action remains of interest, and goes back to the transference. Narcissism can be used in the therapy hour as a series of shifting identifications by the therapist with the possible subjectivities of the patient. The narcissistic satisfaction resides in the mastery of understanding the other person, but it also requires both losing the self within the self of another while retaining an observing self that can be activated to follow the therapeutic line that is being opened up via the understanding, which in itself is usually therapeutic, but not automatically sufficient. In this case the therapist made the identifications with fear, guilt, anger, and loss, but the identifications with compliance, passivity, and the desire to please lay ahead of her and were not as readily accessible.

#2

From the time the therapist heard the former patient's voice on the phone asking for an appointment until he saw her the next week he was annoyed. She had been in and out of therapy with him over a six year period, and despite his best efforts, she always left just when it seemed they were about to actually see a significant change. He envisioned that she would tell him what great difficulty she was in, that her personal life was still a mess, that she knew she should really work at the therapy, that she was really ready to do it, and then the session would be about to end.

He would ask her if she was really ready to come back on a regular basis.

She would say, oh yes, she was, but she couldn't make an appointment then, she didn't know her schedule, she'd have to call him, if that was okay?

Which of course was not a question because that was the best she could, or would, do.

That indeed was approximately what happened when he did see her, except that as the session was coming to a close he deliberately left enough time so that he could point out what she doing in their relationship. She agreed, but said she had not really thought of it that way, and while unconsciously she had not prepared herself for making the next appointment, the current situation was that she really needed to check her schedule, at the moment not with her, and she would indeed call him.

She said, with a little annoyance, "I mean, do you really have to know right now?"

He smiled and said, "No, but it would have been better if you had come prepared to tell me right now."

His annoyance melted a bit. The repetition compulsion was so striking, and so necessary for her to relate. She was quite an orderly, compulsive person, but she often needed to reschedule. The commitment, symbolized in a scheduled appointment, scared her, yet reassured him. The differences between them were numerous, and epitomized in how they were interested in engaging each other. He wanted her to be there, and stay there until she had resolved her chronic difficulty in being with anybody consistently. She wanted to clock in and out, have him be the recyclable parent who would always love her and want to see her when she wanted to see him, but she would not have a mutual relationship with him. In fact, she had no apparent interest in him as a person and in all the time she had known him, she had never asked him a question that could be considered "personal".

His reaction to her comings and goings with him began with a feeling of loss and then started to shift to relief followed by the wish that she would at some point just not return. Thus, this time around he had grown accustomed to being without her. In his ambivalence at her return he was tempted to be difficult, as for example not finding time for her or even questioning her motivation to the point that he believed she would probably back off, at least for another long stretch of time. He also thought of telling her that it just would not work out, that either she, or he, or both of them could not work together in a way that would benefit her. All of these thoughts were quite conscious, and he rejected them as possible courses of action because he did not believe they would benefit her, despite their appeal to him. She had a series of therapists before him, and they always found a way to get rid of her, usually through some reasonable requirement that she found unreasonble. The fact that she had stayed with him for significant lengths of time, that both of them felt progress had been made, and that she kept trying, all argued for continuing to attempt to work with her.

In essence he felt he should not dismiss her or dissuade her because she was dismissive of him. However, his many attempts to illustrate to her through their relationship how she kept people at a distance and made herself difficult to love were met either with defensive explanations or excessive agreements that lacked follow through. Interpretation of these behaviors as transferential brought further agreement, but seemed to be quickly forgotten.

He felt a need to do something about her, and what he was concerned about was being confrontative out of personal annoyance that could easily be rationalized as a therapeutic necessity, but was more likely to be therapeutic for him than for her.

At the same her repetitive unsuccessful behavior in relating to others made the problem quite pointed. So, he asked her, "What is it you want me to do?"

She said, "Well, explain it to me."

He said, "I've done that. You don't get it."

She said, "Of course I don't. It is a terrible thing, but I don't know how to be."

He said, "I want to believe that, because that makes it seem easier, just teach and you can learn, but I don't believe it."

She was surprised. "If I told you, then that's how it must be. I mean, at least that's how it feels to me."

He could feel himself getting calmer as he continued to disagree with her. He said, "No, it doesn't feel that way. I don't know how it feels, but you're not looking, or if you are looking, you are not telling me what you find."

"I'm always honest with you."

"No," he said, "you are not. You cannot be. You sneak the truth in, for yourself as well as for me, but whatever it is, you don't like it."

She said, "You mean I don't like myself much."

"Do you like anybody?"

She was silent. Then, she said defiantly, "Why the hell should I?"

"Then," he said softly, "why should anybody like you?"

"Well", she said quickly "I'm bright, pretty, witty, successful. What's not to like?"

He answered, "That you don't really like the other person."

He was about to go on and illustrate for her how little she liked him, when it struck him that he was afraid to like her.

She said, "I'm afraid to really like somebody. It just means they will go away, die, vanish, hate me forever."

She was echoing his thoughts, but about his feelings towards her. He was patient with her, he was helpful, he would not be easily put off nor would he be manipulated, but he was not about to like her. In fact he has made up his mind never to like her.

He said to her, "I believe you."

Comment

This is a patient that the therapist correctly sensed would present him with the problem of Kernberg's narcissists, particularly disregard for him, as well as Kohut's narcissists, particularly demands for admiration and support. His reaction to her was that unless she changed fundamentally, he at least, would not really like her. He was even somewhat amused that even when she was likeable, he remained indifferent. Other people seemed to like her for a while, until her real self became more apparent, and he actually seemed to like her as well, but he did not in a very fundamental sense. He appreciated certain qualities about her, including her determination and her spontaneity, but he saw the core and refused to touch it because it seemed deadly.

Of course there are people who are fascinated with people who do not like them, but he was never one of them, nor was that necessary here. He just had to be open to her, and his narcissism would not let him. He had categorized her as someone who suffered such emotional abuse as a child that no one could ever make up for it. As a result she schemed her way through relationships, always seeking the other for what he or she could give to her, and using whatever currency that was necessary, money, sex, interest, to create initial attractions to her. Then her enormous hunger for love and attention would increase markedly and the other person would retreat in fear, leaving her bewildered. He must have doubted she would ever change that pattern enough to satisfy him, although he thought it possible that somebody else might like her enough to overlook or deny her demands. She was an object lesson for the therapist as to how to avoid getting caught in a bad relationship, but as a result he held something back. He was afraid, and she was afraid, so they stayed further apart than they had to.

The realization that he would not get enmeshed let him consider the possibility that he could get more attached without losing himself, or her. He could feel his own object hunger along with hers, as well as recognize the distinctions between them. He had been so afraid she would devour him he never truly let her try. He was not indifferent to her nor did he dislike her. In fact, he wanted her to recognize him, but had been unwilling to take his chances with her. He could identify with her pain without feeling it would be his forever.

In this case, the therapist's awareness of his narcissism went in horizontal and vertical directions. At first he liked her, then found her frustrating and annoying, and then developed an apparent indifference to her. The last feeling resulted in his maintaining a certain therapeutic stance towards her, which although flexible, was firm in its insistence on the value of her reality adaptation. His view, made clear to her, was that while she had the option to behave as she liked, there were negative consequences to many of her actions and the historical evidence was available as validation. In their relationship, for example, she could operate in a sporadic fashion, but he remained insistent on the need for consistency to affect more significant change. This stance was sufficiently confrontative, along with interpretations, that he felt he was doing his job without also using her behavior as a way to retaliate against her impersonal treatment of him. The anger was an issue because moving vertically he was becoming more aware of layers of resentment towards her pathological narcissism. This awareness was accompanied by growing consciousness that he feared the impact she was having on him, that he thought more frequently prior to sessions about how to deal with her, how to master the situation with this woman so that it gained meaning, and thus it appeared to him, how to hold her. All this effort and interest was being devoted to a woman he had convinced himself he had neutralized.

The issue here is not what he should have felt, or should have done with what he believed he was feeling, but that he was intent on protecting himself from danger without realizing it, and in doing so, he was making himself anxious to the point of denial. He could not fully experience what it was like to be with her in a session because he would not. Her attitude of exploitation helped him defend himself because it was so prominent. It began to occur to him that if they ever got to have a significant degree of mutuality, or at least if she began to offer that possibility, he would be uncertain as to what to do with it. The fact that he felt more comfortable with her when he was disagreeing with her he now saw as a further defense against his fear of her. He had been in control for that time, but now he recognized how people became afraid of her and wanted to retaliate, and what a problem that must be for her.

His narcissism enlarged to temporary identification with both her rage at not being loved by people she felt she loved, such as her mother, and her fear that she could never do what was involved in mutual loving without being devoured herself by the other person, a feeling she often had when she even heard her mother's voice.

#3

The patient said to her, "I notice that you haven't said much today. Are you feeling all right?"

The therapist was startled. She had actually been thinking of what she had to do when the patient left, which was to pick up one of her children at school. So, was she feeling all right? Yes, and then, no, because she had not been feeling as though she wanted to pay attention, which of course, she reminded herself, was her job.

The patient went on asking, "I hope you're not offended by me asking?"

The therapist said, "Did you want me to say more?"

"No," the patient said, "it is just that, well it seemed to me, even when I came in you were, well kind of distracted, and, well, that's not you. I mean maybe you were ill."

The therapist had not been distracted then, but she had quickly become that way. The patient was talking about work, really the particulars of her job more than her feelings, although the intensity of the way she was speaking revealed that she had strong feelings of being overworked and not appreciated for her efforts.

The therapist played with the idea, if the patient is telling me something that does not interest me, does she deserve my attention? She decided yes, based on the idea that the patient was not required by the therapeutic contract to be interesting for the therapist. The answer seemed obvious enough but she was intrigued that she had asked herself the question. She told herself, the question ought to be , why did you not let yourself stay with the patient?

She asked the patient, "Were you feeling here as you do at work, that you were giving a lot and it was not being appreciated?"

The patient protested, "I don't think so. I know you care about me. It's just that you were different, and I thought you might not be feeling all right, and I was concerned."

The therapist said, "I appreciate your concern. I'm feeling fine, but I'm pretty sure you felt I was not really being with you."

"Well yes," the woman said, "but I didn't think it's because you don't appreciate me."

It was clear to the therapist that she could shift the situation away from the reality of what had occurred by either assigning her own silence to the idea that she had been listening so intently that she did not consider it useful to say more, or consider that the patient was concerned about the loss of the therapist, so she had raised the issue of her possible illness. The latter was undoubtedly true and may well have been brought up even if the therapist had not been distracted, but the point remained that the therapist had let the patient slip away, had dissociated from her.

The therapist thought that it was more important to explore the dissociation with the patient. She asked, "Could it be that at times, when I'm with you, I don't want to listen to you?"

The patient was quiet for a moment. Then she said, "It could be. There are times when I'm with me that I don't want to listen to me either."

"Was this one of those times?"

"You know," she said, "I was afraid to talk about what was really on my mind, and I was boring myself until I figured you'd intervene."

"You wanted me to know what you had in mind?"

"Yes, you know you often do."

The therapist had hesitated to explore what was happening between them because she faulted herself for missing what was happening with the patient.

Beyond that, she realized that she at other times had tuned out this patient because it felt to her as though this patient insisted on being uninteresting. She had refused to see this device of the patient's as a defense because she felt the patient ought to treat her differently, that they had worked together for two years and that there should be an open level of discourse that would eliminate this type of defensiveness. In fact the therapist prided herself on being someone in whom patients found it easy to confide in , to really say what they felt when they felt it. This therapist was the holding environment, and she had just let the baby fall.

"What is it that you did have on your mind?"

"That I'm sick of being dependent on you. I have to say this, I suppose, but I wanted you dead, for a little while, anyway."

The therapist smiled. "Well, I suppose I was, back there in the beginning of the session. How did it feel?"

"Not so good, " said the patient. "I mean, I am dependent, that is how it is."

"What frightens you about the dependency?"

"It sounds paradoxical, but that you'll die, and then there will be no one. I mean, I've been alone so much of my life. I have a husband who is buried in a bottle, and a daughter who hates me. I'm alone."

The therapist said, "I feel we were both alone for a time in this session, and sometimes that happens between us. I wonder about this 'being alone.' What is it that is so troubling about it?"

The patient was crying. After a while she said to the therapist, "I sometimes want to be alone, even when I'm with you. But, what's so bad is when I don't want to be lonely, and I am. No matter what I want, or who I am with, I feel alone when I don't want to be. That's what's bad about it."

The therapist herself suddenly felt alone, although she had not wanted to be. She said to the patient, "I have it."

They sat together for a while in silence together, alone.

Comment

In this case the therapist has altered the symmetry of the relationship with the patient to the point that she expected the patient to keep her interest. In addition, she viewed herself as creating an environment with the patient where the patient would always be forthcoming in a direct way that would provide material that would be stimulating to the therapist. The therapist set the stage and the patient was to be the entertainer, but the therapist also appeared to have written the script and when the patient deviated from it the therapist became disinterested. The disinterest was something that had happened before but it wasn't until the patient commented on the therapist's behavior, that the therapist took notice.

It was also true that usually the therapist behaved in an involved, caring way with this patient, and it was the contrast that caused the disruption. Thus the therapist was accurate in her impression of herself as creating a holding environment, but she denied the limitations in it. She wanted to see the patient's receptive, obsessive discourses as a character trait, a way to lock into herself and lock others out without the others being able to get away, rather than a defense against any current anxiety. It may well have been both a character defense and a reaction to a current feeling, but when the therapist thought about dealing with the patient's alleged concern about the therapist's health, the therapist was feeling guilty about her lapse of attention. She then focused on what she should do about herself, again partially discounting the needs of the therapist.

At the same time, the therapist was very quickly processing what was happening to her, and carefully exploring what she guessed the patient was really concerned about, namely the loss of the therapist. The therapist feels stuck here with having made a basic mistake, namely ignoring the patient, but the therapist is adroit enough to try to find ways to turn the error into a therapeutic advantage. Actually getting distracted, or being bored, or not liking what the patient is saying to the point that the therapist stops hearing the patient, are relatively common episodes during some sessions in any course of therapy, for most, if not all therapists. (I hypothesize all, but, hey, you never know).

Such distractions are clearly not ideal, but they can be useful in terms of providing some clues as to the nature of the transactions taking place between the parties involved, and the state of mind of each. The therapist here was rapidly aware of the need to explore her own reactions. This led to her questioning to herself whether the patient deserved the attention of the therapist, and to the idea that she was feeling rejected by the patient and was angry at the patient, who in turn, now might well get angry at the therapist, particularly if the therapist admits that she was not paying attention to the patient. She saw herself as someone who was not retaliatory and beyond that as someone who the patient would not have a reason to get angry with because the therapist would never give her one. In this process the therapist eradicated the negative transference, and then further surprised herself by giving the patient something to be annoyed about. It turned out the patient had been angry with the therapist anyway, before the session, and the therapist had not seen it because it did not fit her image of herself, or other patients, or of their relationship.

Once the patient's feelings are apparent the therapist is able to change her perspective. Thus at the end of the segment described there is a projective identification where the therapist becomes a container for the patient's loneliness. At this point there is a narcissistic identification with the patient through a painful affect, whereas prior to this, when the patient was a way the therapist did not like, she disowned the patient. The way the session began was with the boring patient and the interesting (but not interested) analyst, in a selective holding environment where the mother-therapist would secretly retaliate if the patient-child would fail to keep the mother's interest. As the therapist's narcissism becomes understandable and apparent to her, she is able to make a shift in her attitude and feelings. As a result the way the segment of the session ends is that the therapist is willing to hold whatever the patient offers, and allows herself to, for the moment, identify with the patient to the point that she experiences an unwanted, unexpected loneliness that she got from the patient. I consider this a transitory narcissistic identification in which the therapist is the patient, yet retains a sense of herself as the therapist as well.

This view of narcissism for the therapist is one that includes empathic linkage, being a selfobject, and intersubjectivity, but also retains a sense of self as agent. Whatever the therapist is doing, and whatever is happening to the therapist, it is motivated by a personal perspective that considers the behavior to be in the person's best interest. In this case the unwanted feeling of loneliness that becomes the therapist's is part of what she considers the best way to be a therapist, and that is her goal. When she was not attending to the patient that was a form of pathological narcissism in which she was taking some immediate gain at the risk of failing to meet her goal, although at the time she did not recognize the situation that way. Instead she thought she was successful enough being as if she was a good-enough therapist, but she was not. Healthy narcissism therefore requires continued reappraisal to keep the self in harmony. The failure of the self to be adaptive and flexible becomes the pathology of narcissism. One does what one does because one is "that kind of a person," which in turn is the embodiment of a personal ideal that is only met part of the time, but which remains always sought after, even if the specifics shift from time to time.

#4

The patient said, "Well, I won't be coming for a while, a month maybe."

The therapist felt uncomfortable, a sense of loss beginning to develop even as he said, "Oh."

"Yeah," said the patient. "This is too much. I could keep doing this forever. I have to learn to handle things on my own."

The therapist protested, "You have only been coming for a short time, and you are improving."

"Sure," said the patient, "I'm improving, but so what, I'm still anxious. What's a little improvement given what I have to deal with."

The therapist could feel his own anger and resentment at this man who often arrives in states of near terror, and who drains the therapist, yet was now depreciating the therapist's efforts. He had found this patient demanding from the start with anxiety compulsively bubbling forth. He was drawn to the man's neediness as well as the associations to his own father's helplessness about which he had been able to do little. Now he had sensed a second chance, and the rather dramatic lessening of anxiety during sessions had been gratifying. At the same time he recognized that beneath the anxiety or wrapped all around it, was a weakened character structure. This man was afraid of everything and everybody, defending against his inadequacies by either running away or becoming antagonistic to the point that he drove others away, leaving him feeling abandoned and continually on the fringe of any interpersonal world.

The therapist thought about his own need to be connected to this man, or more accurately, to get this helpless father connected to him and he also thought about the man's inability to connect, the need to run, to interrupt whatever was forming between them, and then he spoke.

"Why would you want to stop now?"

"Listen, why, why, I mean, I can't do this forever."

The therapist continued to feel annoyed. He both resented and expected this type of response, had seen examples of it in previous sessions, but both anger and disappointment pulled at him to the extent that he found himself struggling to remain sufficiently calm so he could continue his inquiry. He also thought that it could be a relief to let this man go, that indeed they might end up in some kind of perpetual struggle that would be notable primarily for its sadness.

The therapist said, "You haven't been coming forever, nor have you been asked to. You are making progress, but you still have issues to deal with."

"Of course I have issues. I'll always have issues. It's time for me to do something on my own. If I need you I'll call you. Enough of this."

The patient sounded angry, dismissive. At first the therapist experienced it as contempt, but then he wondered what the patient wanted him to do, so he asked.

The patient seemed deflated and confused. He said, "I don't know. I come, I talk, I'm still anxious. Less anxious I'll admit. I know I'm doing better. Being here helps me, but so does an Advil if I have a headache. I can't take one every time my head hurts."

"You might take too many?"

The patient laughed. He said, "It's me, me, me. I'm always needy. I've always been needy. You I'm going to do without, and that's that."

The patient's ambivalence was palpable. It now felt to the therapist as if the patient wanted to be argued into coming, perhaps even shouted down and buried beneath the weight of his pathology that indeed could be cited by the therapist as convincing evidence of the need to continue.

Moving a bit in that direction the therapist asked, "Do you want us to have an argument?"

"God," the man said loudly "I might, I could. I'm always arguing, but so what? I'm a mess."

The man began to cry. The therapist felt curiously detached. Whatever the details of the mess, he did not want to be caught up in it. The man seemed unreal to him, with shoulders moving up and down as he now sobbed. The therapist thought of the man as a puppet, and as a puppet master as well, sometimes voluntarily pulling his own strings, and then losing control, with the strings still being pulled, but now in terrible, diverse ways. The therapist felt a fear that it was happening to him, the pulling of strings, and he thought about just cutting the strings.

He wanted to be free of this string-puller. It could be easy, he thought. I'll tell him, yes, go and think. Try it for yourself. When the man calls again, and it seemed probable that he would, the therapist would have gained the perspective of space and the passage of time. He could start fresh, renewed, and get it right.

The man became calmer. He said, "I'll come back. I'll be here next week at this time."

The therapist said, "I wish we had more time today to discuss what is happening."

"Could I stay?"

The therapist smiled a bit ruefully, and said, "No, I'm afraid not. Someone else is coming soon. But, next week, same time, this time, we will do it next week."

The man stood up. He said, "I know I have to go , but sometimes, it is just the time you know, just the right time."

The therapist could feel the string being pulled, feel his own tension, sense the reprimand, the opportunity that was being offered with the implication that it well could be missing next week. Now the therapist wanted it, when just moments earlier he had felt eager to be rid of the man. Instead he now envisioned a kind of redemption, a reward for the patience and fortitude, the great empathic moment, perhaps symbolized even in a long-term commitment. It was there, and he let it go. He knew better. Besides inconveniencing his next patient with a delay, he doubted the effectiveness of seizing this moment in the way being proposed by the patient. Theirs would be a long struggle, he thought, with many windows of opportunity, opening, closing, opening again.

He said to the man, "Next week, that will be the time."

"All right," said the patient, "and thanks."

Comment

This patient has always been a drain on the therapist's self-esteem. The patient made progress, but his way of asserting himself often showed no regard for the therapist's needs or feelings. Often he seemed to treat the therapist as though he was an Advil to be swallowed, used up, spit out, or just kept on a shelf. He challenged the therapist, particularly in the widespread nature of his distorted ways of protecting himself. The patient's pathological narcissism and angry terror were very compelling in their ability to get the therapist's attention. A the same time there was some scent of the repulsive, some warning that this was someone the therapist had best let go of, not thinking of separation as permanent, but hoping it would just go that way.

Upon reflection, his ambivalence about the patient and the patient's ambivalence about him were associated with his ambivalence about his father. He had always wished he could rescue his father, make him stronger and more powerful, particularly in reference to his mother, whom they both saw as strong, powerful, and devastatingly critical. The patient was married to a woman who supported him for the price of periodic, continual destruction. Thus there was the appeal to the therapist's grandiosity, this patient who so needed his strength that the therapist believed he could indeed overlook, bypass, tolerate, even endure the pulling of his strings. The therapist would meet it with empathic attunements, honed from misattunement. However, these attunements led in the direction of recognizing that in his frequently tormented states the patient could only take, and even that would at times be done begrudgingly. Giving was infrequently there, and the narcissistic ambivalence was the continual background, with the denial of long-term connection rather prominent.

Essentially, it pained the therapist to be involved with the partial reincarnation of his father. He was always failing in his rescue attempts, yet he felt he had to persist. He could feel the connection, he could take note of the sometimes recognition of the value of his presence, and he could even entertain the possibility that when the patient said "thanks," he meant it. Or did he?

That type of question points to the issue of constancy with this patient. He has relied heavily on using his indecision, his abusive questioning, to create enough doubt and ultimately terror to allow him repeatedly to give up. He expects his therapist to give up as well, and provides cause, offers opportunities, but never quite shuts the door. He is the challenge that appeals to the narcissism of many therapists, because he knows he has problems, knows he needs help, feels a connection, makes progress, works, but always threatens to bolt. This patient had a few therapists before this one, and gave them each about a year, but then, usually with their blessing, he departed, the challenge still really in place.

The therapist goes through a series of strong affective reactions as he shifts perspectives. He has continually had difficulty feeling constancy from the patient in a complete fashion. It has always been as though they were both part-objects, and therefore, partially connected. At first the therapist is surprised and disappointed that the patient wants to leave, because the therapist's primary perspective has been to work at fixing this man, particularly by serving as a container and consistent presence for the patient's dependency and fragmented self. Yet while doing this, the therapist has experienced an uncomfortable enmeshment, a reliving of some of his own life with his father where he tried to provide some unwavering support, only to waver as his father would desert him. Thus he also expected the patient to depart, in essence saying the therapist's efforts were insufficient because the patient was beyond repair. The patient, and his father used the excuse of their limited selves to leave the therapist without their support, but with the lingering, renewable memory of their unrelieved suffering.

At one point the therapist shifts his perspective to indifference and a desire to avoid the entanglement, and as he does so the patient makes an offering of himself. He will return. The therapist sees the opening, and moves into it, but with qualifications, namely their interaction needs to be discussed. He establishes a control with the patient that he did not have with his father, and in so doing, differentiates the patient from his father.

The patient then offers immediate gratification, but the narcissism that invited the need to follow the patient's every move is now replaced by conviction about the boundaries of the relationship. The therapeutic frame now begins to fit.

Overview

The therapist's role in terms of expressing healthy narcissism is to be effective with the patient, requiring a focus on getting the task accomplished. The therapist's role in terms cf expressing pathological narcissism becomes a defensive satisfaction of a personal need under the guise of therapeutic effectiveness. The degree of pathology is variable, and the type of narcissism being expressed by the therapist is subject to rather frequent, probably inevitable oscillations. In that vein we can consider what happens as examples of the "psychopathology of everyday life," to be expected and actually capable of facilitating life's endeavors through increased understanding. Narcissism is not pathological because it is subjective, for, as Renik (1993) notes, analytic technique is always subjective. Narcissism becomes pathological in sessions when the work shifts to a focus on the therapist's needs in such a way that the patient's needs are neglected. Therapeutic effectiveness then requires the analyst to note the changes in focus and discern ways to shift the focus back to using the self as a therapeutic instrument. Throughout, however, the therapy is always a personal, narcissistic activity for the analyst, who along with the patient, has capacities for self-deception that are part of narcissism and require continual scrutiny.

In the first example, the therapist wants the patient to be a certain way that would make her feel most comfortable. She wants the patient to identify with her but she becomes aware of her negation of the patient's autonomy, and she allows herself to make a shift and identify with parts of the patient. Originally she tries to satisfy a personal need for bonding and partial merger by pulling the patient in to a part of herself, but she becomes aware of the poor fit. As a result she satisfies the same need for connection, but by refocusing the identification. All the while her internal forces are key determinants for what takes place.

In the second example the analyst seeks a way to develop a level of comfort with the patient and settles on indifference. However, he then becomes aware of the ineffectiveness of such an approach, and its defensive nature. He realizes how great an impact she actually does have on him, how he is afraid to engage yet would actually like to be more connected, and then he shifts his focus. In so doing he also achieves a greater level of comfort in being with her, thus satisfying the original narcissistic need.

In the third example the therapist has deceived herself into believing that the patient is unaware of an ongoing disinterest on the therapist's part. The deception is motivated by the need to symbolize the holding environment at its most magnificent regardless of contrary or discrepant feelings. When these appear the analyst drifts away without registering the drift and its possible impact. However, when the therapist allows herself to see how she's moving away from the patient, she is able to process her feelings and move back to the holding position that she usually, but not eternally maintained. In this resolution she has a better understanding of both herself and her patient, and that is more of what she wanted than she was getting by her previous attempts at narcissistic satisfaction.

In the final example the therapist has a need to rework his relationship with his father so that he gets his father to stay with him as an ongoing presence. His focus is on rescuing the patient and being rewarded with recognition, and he is shocked when the patient pulls away. At first he focuses on the narcissistic injury in the apparent rejection by the patient, but as he looks into the details of this rejection his view begins to shift. He starts to see the patient in a more differentiated light, and he is able to be more therapeutic. At the same time, the reworking of his relationship with his father continues but in a way that does not exploit the patient.

The negative consequences of using pathological narcissism in countertransferential enactments has been well documented (Schwaber, 1992). Here we stress the positive developments arising from the analyst's subjectivity. The analyst and the patient are each providing interpretations of reality and fantasy. Therapeutic progress then takes place through a dialectical interaction of these personalized viewpoints. We will next consider how a similar process takes place in supervision.

Supervisory Sessions
#1

The supervisee states, "I asked the patient what was happening when she told me on the phone that she didn't feel like talking to me. She said that's how it is. There are days like that when she just doesn't want to see me."

The supervisor asked, "What did you say?"

"At first I didn't know what to say, she said it so definitively."

The supervisor feels a bit impatient. The supervisee continues.

"Then I told her, well, something must be troubling you when that happens. That's when you really need to come in. She said, I know. I felt that way today so I came in."

"The patient said, 'I know'?"

"Yes."

"How did that make you feel?"

"I was glad she came in."

The supervisor continues to feel impatient. She tells the supervisee, "Let's think about her telling you she already knew what you were telling her. The patient may be defensive, preventing you from giving her an insight."

"I didn't think of her as being defensive. I mean, I suppose she was, but I was just glad she came."

The supervisor is aware that she is trying to create an area of interest, namely the interaction between the patient and the therapist, but the supervisee has a different emphasis. This has been a pattern in the supervision, as from the supervisor's point of view she and the supervisee are frequently going in different directions, and she feels the supervisee misses some important issues in her travels. She also experiences the supervisee as tentative and uncertain of her autonomy, and the supervisor feels restricted by the supervisee's anxiety.

She decides to pursue the feelings about the patient coming. She asks, "Did you feel you were losing this patient?"

"I don't know, maybe. She usually comes but then there are times when she doesn't. I suppose it worries me then. I mean, that's when I think about it, that perhaps she'll stop."

Again the supervisor feels blocked, and she also feels she is making the supervisee anxious. She feels a mixture of guilt and annoyance, and the guilt appears to win out. She decides to return to the matter of what was troubling the patient. When she asks about that the supervisee appears relieved.

"It was about her boyfriend. He was being difficult, and her mother was telling her, 'I told you he was no good,' and she thought maybe her mother was right, but she didn't want to admit it.

She paused, then continued, "The mother is often critical of what she does, but feels powerless to stop her, or at least, she doesn't really try to stop her."

The supervisor feels the need for clarification. She asks, "How was the boyfriend being difficult?"

"He wanted to have sex with her, and, you know, she's an adolescent. She isn't sure what she wants about sex. Her mother doesn't want her to, and she has been kind of vague with the mother, but she gets the picture."

The supervisor feels as though she doesn't get the picture, or she doesn't like the picture she is getting of the supervisee as a therapist. She asks about the transference.

"How do you feel the patient sees you?"

The supervisee appears uncomfortable and answers quickly, "Different from her mother. Not critical."

The supervisor senses that the supervisee is experiencing her as critical, does not want this to happen, yet appears so anxious that she cannot discuss what is happening to her in the supervision. The supervisor does not like to be criticized herself so she feels more empathy for the supervisee than she had felt up to this point. The phrase, "not critical," resonates for her.

She asks, "What helps you in being not critical?"

"Well, I mean, I know it's not therapeutic. I mean, not how therapists are supposed to be, but it's more than that for me. I would not want to have a critical mother either."

"So you think that the patient may sense this, that she can feel you are on her side?"

"Yes. I mean, when she doesn't come she may have doubts, but the rest of the time I feel she knows I am different from her mother."

"She trusts you."

"Yes, I mean, not that much I suppose, because she is not very trusting, but more than her mother who just complains about her behavior but doesn't stop her or help her, just complains."

Comment

The supervisor has an agenda here. She is particularly interested in getting the therapist to talk about and understand her relationship with the patient. She would also like to go beyond that to the supervisor-supervisee relationship because she considers that a key feature in teaching the supervisee to be a more effective therapist. However, the supervisee appears to prevent her from taking the first step, and in the prevention process sends a message that the supervisor experiences as a warning that getting into their relationship will not be constructive. Instead, the supervisee appears content-and-patient-focused. The transference and the resistance are briefly noted, as is the countertransference, but there is no voluntary exploration. The therapist appears aware of their existence, but diminishes their existence. All of this frustrates the supervisor and causes her to diminish the value of the supervisee. This dimunition is reinforced by the supervisee's anxiety. She has a hesitant style, and it is clear that the supervisor's style is making her more uncomfortable.

The supervisor surmises the presence of a parallel process, but views it as if she was making the supervisee anxious and probably the supervisee does not want to be with her in the same way the patient does not want to see the therapist. So at first the supervisor views the therapist as lacking empathy for the patient, because she hypothesizes that the supervisee is too busy trying to contain her anxiety about relating to the patient. Thus the therapist is making the patient anxious akin to the supervisor making the therapist anxious.

When the supervisee begins to talk about the patient's mother the supervisor hears this as further avoidance. Now she believes that the supervisee wants to take still another step away from the patient-therapist relationship. At the same time, the supervisor's image of herself as a caring, concerned person who is very adept at relating to others is suffering a narcissistic injury. She is not able to get the supervisee to relate to her in a helpful, useful way. She feels guilty, fearing that she had made the supervisee afraid of her and afraid of dealing with the patient. She believes that the supervisee is partially the cause of the state of affairs, and she is partially the cause, with the result that she is confused and conflicted as to what to do herself, yet still does not feel connected to or identified with the supervisee. Instead, despite her discomfort with herself, she feels too much of a difference from the supervisee to bridge the gap.

Her perspective starts to shift when the supervisee uses the words, "not critical." She develops an interest in the supervisee through the understanding of their mutual aversion to criticism, and to critical mothers. She starts to see a different version of parallel process in which she has played the role of the patient's mother, less overtly critical but disapproving none the less, and not helpful. The supervisee is placed in a position of uncomfortable autonomy where she gets the impression of doing the wrong thing in both therapy and supervision. She cannot explain herself directly and openly because she is working in a way that appears too different from what would interest the supervisor. The supervisor realizes she is not taking a sufficient look at the supervisee to either understand her or find a way to successfully encourage her to better depict her functioning as a therapist.

With this realization the supervisor begins to enlarge her perspective. She moves toward the strength of the supervisee, namely acceptance of the patient, validates it, and gives the supervisee a reason to use that strength with her. The supervisee responds to this by indeed telling her more so that the rationale for working with the patient starts to get clarified.

It is possible that the supervisor might have worked out their differences by talking directly about the issue, but it is also possible that the supervisee would have increased her defensiveness to the point of denial. The supervisor now has a way to teach and the supervisee to learn. The obstacle was not so much the supervisor's method as her view of herself as having an approach to supervision that was destined to be effective regardless of the limitations in her comprehension of the supervisee. She saw the supervisee as too different from herself. Once she made a connection, instead of insisting the supervisee do it, they began to work together without either being the critical reproachful mother that both of them had found discomforting.

#2

The supervisor said to her, "You are working well with this patient, but I don't get much of a feel for you, for who you are in this supervision, and really in the therapy process."

"I know," she said.

She paused. He did not say anything.

She continued. "It will come. It just takes time."

He did not want to leave it there. He felt there was a missing ingredient to what was otherwise an effective supervisory process, and she was the ingredient. He felt as if she was not really there. Only a portion of her was there, a categorized person who was very strict about staying in place, yet suffered because of the way she restricted herself.

In turn, he felt that only a portion of him was there as well, and he saw the situation as role exaggeration, supervision and supervise, teacher and student, but not real people. If it continued this way he would feel controlled, limited, and disregarded because he felt she was doing that to him in her own way and he needed to break through it, either by understanding more of its origin, or having the pattern change.

He asked her, "Why does it need it need to take time?"

She said, "I would like to be more open about myself with you. I think it would be valuable, for me as a person, and for me as a therapist, but I feel you already know about me."

He was puzzled. He said, "I know you are bright, have talent as a therapist, but I don't know about you. I'd like to, I'm open to it, but I don't know."

"Look," she said, "It isn't you. It's me."

He smiled. "You could tell that I was concerned that I was limiting you in some way?"

She smiled. "Yes, but that's not it. It is because you are friends with my former supervisor, and I know she told you about me, about my situation, about what has happened to me. She told me she told you. I was always talking to her. I just talked too much to her, and she talked too much to other people. I mean, she told me about it, as though I had given her permission, and as though it would be helpful to me. She even said it would be good if you knew, that you were very understanding, but I don't want to talk about myself anymore. Perhaps I should, but I'm just getting by this way, and that is it, I just want to get through this institute."

She was distraught, frustration and desperation in her tone. He felt annoyed at the other supervisor, who did gossip and indeed had attempted to talk to him about the supervisee. However, he had politely directed the conversation in a different direction. He had known then that he was going to supervise her and he did not want to have information about her that did not come from her. He believed he worked better with someone when he formed his views and opinions as the supervision proceeded.

He said to her, "It is very possible that your former supervisor talked to me about you, but, although we are friends, I did not really listen. It just was not the way I wanted to get to know you."

He could tell she did not completely believe him. She said, "I know you try to be objective, but you know I had, probably still have, a personal problem, and I feel as if you are just waiting for me to tell you how that affects my work, and it probably does, I mean I can't stand loss so I'll either hang on to patients, or beat them to it and convince them they should terminate. Still, I don't want to talk about it, now anyway. I will, I know I even want to."

He felt her ambivalence, as well as his own. He wanted her to confide in him, to trust him, to recognize him as indeed the understanding person the other supervisor had said he was, but he wasn't interested in her openness for the sake of discovering her secret or really, from her viewpoint, hearing more about it, the current version. His style as a supervisor was direct, trying to ascertain a complete picture. In particular he did not want to be identified as the former supervisor.

He said, "I want to know you, not it, or only it to the extent that you are it. And I don't really try to be objective. I know I'm subjective, as we all are. I do try to be helpful, to not get in the way, to listen. I know more about you now than I did before."

She smiled. "You know what I don't want to do."

"Yes, and I know what that feels like, to not want to do."

"Oh," she asked, "what is it you don't want to do?"

"I don't want to talk about this anymore, " he said, "but, I do want to know how you feel about having this discussion."

She laughed.

Comment

This supervisor has a need to confront, to get to what he sees as an issue and have it discussed, yet he is working with someone who has a need to conceal, even if she believes that what is concealed could be affecting her work as a therapist. At the same time, she is mindful of countertransference, but wants to work out various significant aspects of it for herself. The supervisor can feel this, and disagrees with her approach to the extent that her prefers she utilize him in the process.

She accepts him as a helper, but limits the areas of help she will request, or take if it is offered. He finds that frustrating, and is straightforward about the degree to which he experiences her as being hidden. He is telling her, in this experience you are avoiding me, and you act as if you want me to avoid you. The supervision has been contained in the realms of technique and theory primarily, thereby depersonalizing it. Her remark about his own objectivity disturbs him and he refutes it immediately. He does not even qualify his subjectivity that much, although in practice he has no intention of letting personal needs interfere with the supervision. He is trying to get that message across to her, that who she is has a significance to him and for the work that should not be avoided. She agrees, sort of, but she still wants to be avoidant. Her message to him is, yes, but not now.

He is patient. His need is not to know now, or to know a specific event or feeling, but more to tell her what he feels. He does this being aware that it may result in her being anxious and defensive, although he hopes that if she does need to protect herself she will lose the need in talking to him. Even if she does not, he figures that he will have a better sense of her than if he leaves the issue untouched. His tendency is to comment on what he sees, keeping timing and the manner of his comments as significant considerations.

At issue here is, did she want to hear him? It seems as though she did, although she has more of a secret than he thought, and she believes he knew much more. Apparently she was concerned that he would judge her negatively, perhaps see her as limited and vulnerable when she was eager to demonstrate her strength. Her strength came through to him in her work with patients, but it was in her interaction with him that the idea of loss, the "something missing" appeared.

His narcissistic need was to find what was missing, but the object of his search was not what she thought it would be. As his inquiry proceeds he keeps encountering what he doesn't want to know. There is a negative impression of his friend who had been her supervisor, her erroneous belief that he knows things about her because his friend said that she had told him, her probable fusion of him with his friend, and her impression that he is trying to get her to talk about a specific problem. Being this object of her projections brings him in closer touch with his own need for autonomy and allows him to reconsider how he might be viewing her. He does know that his friend was trying to convey to him that she had a personal problem, so he could see her reticence as a way to preserve her autonomy. He is a potential invader whom she believes already knows where she is defenseless but is biding his time before striking. That image of himself, however, is not appealing so he can't just let it sit until she clears it, but he can refocus to the extent that he will ask about her in a very open-ended way.

His approach appears effective. She has her secret in mind, and has a desire to talk about it, but in her time. He discovers that she wants to let him know more about her, as well as why she has held back. He indeed does get to know her better, is able to identify with her reluctance, and learns that she is struggling with separation issues that play a role in how she works with patients.

He also has a need to clarify who he is, so he takes a risk with his comment about his use of subjectivity. He wants to emphasize a mutual recognition of each other as individuals, made apparent as he indicates his empathy for the autonomy that she is asking for. Then, at the end, they both ease the tension before he shifts the specific focus. He is telling her that they now have an area for discussion of both their feelings, namely what has just transpired, instead of her past. This also appears to be congruent with her current feelings.

#3

The supervisee comments, "This guy keeps changing his appointments, and then he doesn't show, and I'm waiting, and I'm annoyed: I feel like I'm always putting out for him and he really doesn't respond."

The supervisor felt unsympathetic and somewhat annoyed, experiencing the supervisee as a complaining child. She asked him, "What are you expecting?"

"More of a commitment, more reciprocity. Maybe I shouldn't, I suppose, but I do."

"Didn't you tell me that this is a major problem for this patient, that he's not responsible?" In asking the question she was aware that she depersonalized the patient-therapist relationship by switching from "commitment" (the therapist's word) to "responsibility."

"Yes, so I suppose I shouldn't expect him to behave differently with me than with anybody else."

"Well, " she said, "this is a man whose parents neglected him, particularly his father, so he is replaying the father-son relationship with you in the transference."

"All right, but I'm being a different father for him than he had."

"I see," she said, "you are providing a corrective emotional experience." She wondered if she had used a sarcastic tone.

The supervisee felt a need to further explain himself. He said, "I don't know whether I would call it 'corrective,' but I believe it is different."

She said, "You're slanting the transference, trying to move it in a particular direction instead of just letting it evolve, letting him project."

He argued with her. "I'm not trying to create a particular type of transference. I'm just attempting to develop a working alliance. I'm being there for the guy and sure that's different from the way his father was, and his mother picked on him, but I'm just doing what I am supposed to be doing."

She felt annoyed. She said, "Well, it isn't working, is it?"

He admitted it was not, but he attributed it to the patient's pathology.

She said, "You have been making some interpretations of the patient's behavior. Perhaps you want to reconsider them."

She was struck by her persistence in trying to teach him an integration of theory with practice, but her avoidance of highlighting his need to get certain responses from the patient as a reward for her efforts.

"I could do that," he said. "Now I have been interpreting mainly around his aggression toward his father, and I suppose he just keeps acting that out."

Her associations were that the supervisee was acting out with her, and that the patient, despite his therapist's efforts, was not experiencing the therapist as a consistent presence. In turn, the supervisee did not experience her as there for him, and he could be joining with the patient in his resistance to supervision. The patient played a testing game with the therapist, who responded with interpretations and felt no gratitude in return. The therapist then tested her, and she responded with rather critical theoretically-based explanations, and certainly felt no gratitude from him. However, she did notice he was more comfortable with her suggestion of switching the interpretive focus than any of her other comments, but she did not consider the interpretations the major issue. She wanted to keep the focus on the content of his sessions because she felt more comfortable in a less affective, personalized realm. Otherwise, she thought, I will attack this man for his attitude toward the patient, and more than that, his attitude about me.

"Let's rethink this," she said. "Let's hypothesize that the patient, although he likes you, is afraid to show it because while you may appear to be different than his father, you won't be. He is afraid it will be a repeat."

"Yes," said the supervisee, "that could be. I mean, I believe he does like me, but it certainly could be that I'm expecting him to just trust me when he needs more time to just check me out."

"So," she said, "you could consider that paradoxically if you felt less consistent, if you liked him less, he might even like you more."

"You mean then I would be more like his father."

"Yes," she said, "and he could respond with anger but he could also respond by trying to get you to love him by trying to do whatever it is he thinks you want."

"It's funny," the supervisee said, "I thought you were implying that I didn't really like this guy, but now I get the idea that even if I do like him, and he likes me, his dynamics are such that he needs to keep testing me."

She said softly, "I want to help you understand this patient as fully as possible."

Now she was aware that she had become more personal, breaking her reserve and less concerned about her anger. She had not been looking for gratitude, but for an alliance of understanding and perhaps the supervisee could have a similar goal. She had wanted him to become stronger through knowing more, and she began to feel he could be open to that.

He said, "You know I kept feeling frustrated, I put so much emphasis on being there for the guy, and why should he be there for me? He is not there for anybody, I suppose because he is so afraid."

"So," she said, "I have a feeling we could take a look at that, you know, dealing with somebody who wants to be there but is afraid. Not such an easy person to be with, for anybody."

"Yes," he said, "but I want to make this work, the therapy."

"I believe you do," she said.

Comment

In this case the supervisor initially dislikes the supervisee. She sees him as weak and incompetent, and he reminds her of people in her life who were like him. They angered her and she showed it, often to her own regret. The possibility of repeating that preoccupies her in the supervision so she attempts to avoid the relationship between them and instead uses the content of the therapy sessions to teach the supervisee how to conduct the therapy.

Her customary supervisory style is in this vein, namely putting the emphasis on what is happening between the therapist and patient, as well as on her impressions. The superviser-supervisee relationship and the therapist's countertransference are not stressed. In this case her usual approach is even more attractive to her because of her disdain for the supervisee. However, she is aware of her feelings and does not want them to obstruct the supervision. She realizes that her trenchant comments, such as the "corrective emotional experience," are not greeted with appreciative insight. She realizes that it is not only the therapy that is not working, but the supervision as well. Her efforts are as fruitless as his.

She could continue to pathologize the supervisee. She wants to keep a distance from him as though she fears that his emotional state will be catching. She is taken back by his direct description of his frustration with the patient and his apparent need for gratitude, or even mutuality. She wants to view herself as different from the man, to keep clearly separated and individuated at all times. She does not want to show her negative feelings that much because that would be too much of an engagement with him, but she definitely has an edge in her comments. Also, while he is often defensive with her and feels the unstated pressure, he does contest her and is willing to engage her.

What eventually causes her to shift perspectives is her growing awareness of her ineffective role in the situation. She sees his role, both with the patient and with her, and she sees his reluctance to look at his own motives, and that leads her to question her own way of operating. The supervisee may be misunderstanding the patient, but she may be misunderstanding the supervisee. When she hears his willingness to reconsider his interpretations she begins to think about how she can help him. She also realizes that prior to that she would have considered what she was doing as trying to be helpful, but self-protection was more of her issue.

As her fear of contagion dissipates, she feels less hostility toward the supervisee. She can personalize her comments more easily, make it their endeavor rather than staying so separate. She does not become dramatically different, she does not start to openly focus on the relationship between them, but she becomes interested in developing more of a holding environment for the supervisee, and he appears responsive to her efforts. Her view of what supervision should emphasize does not change, but her impression of the supervisee is altered. As part of the change she can shift her style, allow herself to be more a part of what is happening between them without overtly discussing their relationship. Her narcissism is no longer the potential danger for him, and in the way he is now reacting to her, it is not dangerous for her either.

She has neutralized a considerable amount of her aggression and then redirected it in the service of developing a more productive way to work with the supervisee. She has shifted her method of mastering the situation from using pointed questions that tended to unbalance him, yet protected her, to joining with him in what they are doing. In this shift she remains congruent with her view of the supervisory process, particularly her helpful role in it which is important for her narcissistic satisfaction. Thus the joining with him continues her belief that it is a collaborative relationship focused on the therapist-patient interaction, but not on the supervisor-supervisee relationship. The latter is in her awareness, and it certainly could be addressed given the tension between them, but she considers that less effective than her emphasis. Shifting that emphasis would disturb her narcissistic equilibrium, so she finds a way to ease the tension indirectly. Her need is to work in a way that both suits her and helps the supervisee, and she does find a way to do that.

#4

The supervisee told him, "This woman feels very guilty about having affairs. She's really trying to work things out with her husband."

Her tone seemed to imply that she saw this as a therapeutic goal. The supervisor was somewhat surprised. She was very open in her presentation, often delving into her countertransference and in so doing had left him with the impression that she was very liberal. He had pictured her as someone who would not disapprove of an affair, and in fact would probably consider it fine if the person felt like doing it.

He asked her, "Do you want her to stop having affairs?"

She said, "Well yes. I mean, she is being deceitful, and that's not good."

He felt put off by her use of universals, her unexpected moralizing. He experienced her as changing from a free-spirited sexual liberal to a rather narrow person who just happened not to be married to the person she was living with, and he didn't like the transformation. He felt uneasy in the presence of this new person. In their relationship there had been a relative security of feeling real for him which was prompted by her self-disclosures. Most of this feeling centered around a relief that he could be open with her about his motivations if he so desired. He did not experience either one of them as having a sexual interest in each other, but as capable of being open with each other. Suddenly an area of openness got closed, and with it the whole idea of his openness.

He said to her, "I'm reluctant to say it is good to be deceitful but, put it this way, the truth can be harmful to others in certain circumstances. This woman is concealing something from her husband that could be painful for him to know."

She agreed, but added that she placed great value on fidelity.

He said, "You may, but does she have to?"

She conceded that the patient did not.

He continued, "You can explore with her what her affairs are about, why she is disinterested in her husband, why she's guilty, what she feels about all this."

"I know," she interrupted, "but don't make decisions for her. I just started thinking she really feels guilty, and she wants to try to make everything all right. I started to give it a direction, but a direction I think she wants to take."

"Perhaps, " he said, "but for what reason? Why is she becoming guilty now? She has been having affairs for years. She reports continual unhappiness with her husband. I know she used a type of dissociation to separate herself from her feelings, but why is that no longer effective?"

"You mean she may be getting some kind of a message from me. I could be making her guilty, which I don't really want to do."

"You could be providing a safe place for her to connect with her feelings, including guilt, but because she feels guilty that does not mean she has to take a particular course of action."

He felt this supervisee was quite skilled at providing a safe holding environment, and the patient indeed became very open with her, but now she could be shutting the patient down just as her comments had shut him down. He felt as if he became centered on her relationship with the patient and in turn moved away from a more fluid approach in which he easily slipped into the different relationships available in doing supervision. He found the constriction disrupting, perhaps a type of betrayal given the qualities he had projected into the supervisee.

She said, "You know, that's what happens to me. I get to thinking, this patient is just like me, and she isn't. I like her, and so I want to move her along. I think, well, she is stuck, living with the guy and always feeling she's dishonest, and I wouldn't want to be that way."

"Or be the recipient of it, the one who was fooled?"

"Yes, sure, I wouldn't want to be fooled, but I sense that if she gets confessional he won't like it, and neither will she. She may be getting in that kind of mood, and trying to tell me about what she's thinking of doing."

"Could be. You could find out."

"Yes, I get ahead of myself, or her. It is as though I'm on a roll, things just have to happen, you know what I mean?"

He sensed then that she was reaching out to him for some confirmation that she was all right, or beyond, that they were all right. He wasn't sure if she picked up the distance, or just his possible disapproval. She didn't appear so satisfied with her work, and he could see they were reaching an understanding as to her therapeutic role. He decided to check out the status of their relationship.

He told her, "I didn't expect you to feel so negatively about the patient's sexual behavior. It doesn't seem like you, or at least my image of you."

She told him, "I know what you mean. I get caught up in being one way, you know, honest, and I lose sight of the value of autonomy, or something like that. I'm sounding stilted. It isn't coming out right."

He laughed. "Your honesty is appreciated. It helps me to know what you feel, what directions you are going in. I'm probably pushing a little harder with you than I might otherwise do because you are talented, but I don't want to overwhelm you with insights either."

She said, "What you are doing helps. A lot of the time I'm trying to find myself as a therapist, well, as a person. Sometimes I think I'm there or something, and then it changes, you know?'

"Yes," he said, "I know."

Comment

In this supervision the supervisor is confronted with disappointment as he feels a narcissistic injury that does not appear to be intentional, or even accurate. His supervisory style tends to shift with the supervisee, but he has one style that he finds most appealing. In that mode the attitude of the supervisee is such that she offers the supervisor a large spontaneity zone. He feels free, even if he has no need to exercise the freedom, and as a result he gives the supervisee a special status, although he does not tell her this. He may well be unaware of it until she does something that makes him rethink his impression of her.

The supervisor has a very interactive sense of self, one that can be particularly dependent on selfobjects. At the same time it is a self that remains relatively closed and differentiated unless he feels a particular kinship to the other person. With this supervisee he felt that they had bonded around a type of anti-establishment sentiment that embraced a liberal attitude toward behavior that is often the object of external regulations. His narcissism points him in the direction of fine-tuning with all supervisees, and he enjoys the sense of competence that comes with accomplishing good working relationships. However, he also has a need to be more expressive and irrational than he usually finds possible in the supervisory situation. Thus when he meets a supervisee that seems to be similar to him, a partial twinship transference gets into their relationship. Generally this creates a better supervisory environment for the supervisee as well but has potential liabilities.

In this case he feels that in the beginning he has made an error, and he wants to dissolve the bond between them. The supervisee has also made an error with the patient as well, seeing the patient as her twin, and she also is disturbed by the mistake. Both the supervisor and supervisee feel a loss, but he is positioned so that she can use his interventions to understand what she is doing. In turn, as part of the supervisory process, she can learn to realign her efforts with the patient. Her openness with the supervisor has been well received in the past, and she continues to make use of it, including some rapprochement refueling where she implies and asks for his understanding.

When she does this it becomes more obvious to him that he is the object of his own sensitivity. She is being reactive to her needs in regard to the patient while scarcely aware that he has a need for her to fit the image he has in place. In fact, he begins to see that she is as always trying to maintain her cohesive self of the moment, which remains open to discussions about that very cohesiveness. It is not her intention to prevent him from making any intervention he pleases, but he is threatened by the appearance of differences between them.

The power of the threat is very noticeable to him. He keeps working in the direction that he considers most effective, namely to get the supervisee to reconsider how she is working with the patient, and in the process, to explore the origins of what she is doing. He would have proceeded in this manner regardless of whether he felt disappointed or not. His sense of competence carries him in the session, but he is looking for a way out of a defensive stance that concerns him. He doesn't like feeling restricted where once he felt expansive. He knows he is moving away from her, and he wants to move back.

He makes the change in response to her asking him, "you know what I mean?" It is a reminder to him that she is not going anyplace unless he insists on sending her away. He begins to wonder if her difference of viewpoint is something he must inflict upon himself as dangerous, given that he already accepts other differences between them.

He connects with the original maternal disapproval that engenders such disappointment for him, and he then differentiates her from his mother. The supervisee moves back into place, less of a twin than before but better recognized. As an external object she suddenly supplied the means for destruction of his internalized image, and appeared as a re-creation that was inspired by a different view of the self. His narcissism no longer requires such a drastic defensiveness, either in terms of the relationship to the object, or as an internalization. He becomes able to get at ease with himself as he helps the supervisee to become more open to the patient.

Overview

Therapy often shadows supervision, but in supervision the teacher-student structure is expected. As a result narcissistic security is something the supervisor is more likely to expect than would be the case for the analyst doing therapy. These examples illustrate how that security rests on different expectations for each supervisor. What they share, however, is a desire to be effective using their own style of supervision. When that style is experienced by the supervisors as ineffective the result is both a narcissistic injury and a signal to reconsider themselves in the supervisory session.

The segments of supervision that have been described illustrate the potential downside of countertransference enactments followed by the supervisors' successes in developing a narcissistic equilibrium that facilitates the supervisory process. Eventually they recover from their mistakes by emphasizing the need to be effective. The supervisors, just like the analysts in the therapy examples, are generally focused on their competency. Renik (1993) in describing the constructive role of subjectivity, takes note of the overall conscientiousness of analysts, which in turn serves as a significant component of healthy narcissism.

The trigger for narcissistic imbalance appears in the perception by supervisors of discomforting differences between their supervisees and themselves. Werman (1989) has discussed the impact of such differences in the context of Freud's "narcissism of minor differences" (1917, p.199). Such narcissism is a need to retain distinctiveness, or a need to maintain a bond which is disrupted by the appearance of difference between the self and the other. Thus in some instances a person may feel the loss of distinctiveness, such as a diminution of an established role, whereas in other instances, there can be a loss of connection. The reaction to the differences is often a hostile one as the person feels under attack and struggles to preserve their identity. In the examples given, identity change became an issue but was resolved by narcissistic shifts so that the therapists and supervisors created a new self-equilibrium that reflected perceived changes in their relationships to others as well as in their self relationships.

The emphasis thought this chapter has been on the constructive value of narcissism, manifested in shifting personal perspectives so that the self is satisfied that it is operating in a constructive way. In the examples given this means being an effective analyst or supervisor. At the same time, narcissistic needs could prevail in pathological ways where patients or supervisors are exploited. However, the possibility of exploitation is not eliminated or reduced by disavowing the subjectivity of the analyst or the supervisor. Instead, it is necessary to recognize the different possibilities for narcissism, constructive and destructive, and through specific recognitions continually reevaluate personal perspectives with the aim of maintaining narcissism as a positive force in every situation.

Such recognition and evaluative processing does not always occur, or it occurs in distorted, defensive ways that lead to the allowance and even legitimatizing of exploitations. The intensity of aggression that may flow from narcissistic injuries that appeared in apparently minor differences has been noted by Volkan (1986) as a significant component of hostilities between nations. Hoffman (1983) points out the potential for error in viewing the analyst's view of reality as authoritative as an illustration of distorted narcissism in the analytic situation.

Where are we left then with the issue of when the therapists or supervisors' narcissism becomes pathological? We start with the inevitable presence of subjectivity, and following the recognition, it is necessary to understand the effects, and then to make attempts to maintain narcissism as a constructive characteristic. In essence the upside of narcissism is emphasized while the downside is constrained, keeping in mind the impossibility of always doing the best thing for all concerned. The pursuit of healthy narcissism in analytic endeavors is a continual activity and an incomplete process that despite its frustrations is best carried out in a context of accepting and understanding analysts' personal needs.

". . . our guiding metaphor might be the analyst as skier or surfer - someone who allows himself or herself to be acted upon by powerful forces, knowing that they are to be managed and harnessed, rather than completely controlled" (Renik, 1993,p.565).

VII
Separation and Connection

Introduction

There are two themes that symbolize the evolution of psychoanalytic theory and practice in regard to the development of relationships. Separation is the first, and is prominent in *structural theory* which includes classical drive theory, ego psychology, and the contemporary versions of these theories. Connection is the second, and is prominent in *relational theory* which includes interpersonal, object relations, and self theories. There are significant variations on many issues within the categories, but they are sufficiently accurate portrayals of the major psychoanalytic ways of viewing relationships. Mainstream psychoanalytic thinking has moved from a strong emphasis on separation-individuation to a much broader view of the power of interpersonal relations that emphasizes connections to others. There has been a significant change in focus from individuality and objectivity to mutuality and subjectivity as primary areas of inquiry in both theory and practice. However, despite issues of distinction and opposition, it is not as though one doctrine replaced another, but rather that there are now more viable psychoanalytic viewpoints than there were before, and these different beliefs and practices tend to contain at least some appreciation of each other. Given that narcissism originated as a concept that was already a bit deconstructed, and has gone on to accrue a history of multiple meanings, it is of interest to now look at narcissism in the context of the change in primacy from separation to connection.

Separation

Separation has long been valued as the necessary path to achieving an identity. There is a goal of self-sufficiency that does not bypass dependency, but does emphasize the ability to stand alone if and when that is necessary. Object relations provide the material for the processes of identifications that are used in the formations of self-representations that are differentiated from object representations. Relational environments produce the settings for the emergence of individuation and the development of autonomy which does include a relational stance as, at the very least, an adaptation. Structural theory acknowledges the importance of relational interaction, but emphasizes the developmental goal of internalization of structure to foster independence from others. The personal perspective contained in such an emphasis on individuality highlights drive motivation rather than relational, with separation appearing as more of an ultimate goal than connection. Thus the psychosexual stages which emphasized drive development were eventually accompanied by the stages of separation-individuation (Mahler, Pine, & Bergman, 1975). Also, in discussing the role of the libidinal and aggressive drives, Blanck and Blanck state, "The story of ego psychology is that psychological connections must also be severed in order for the individual to attain an identity" (1994, p.17). These authors also describe a "normal separating thrust" (p. 91).

Although object relations are viewed as more the instruments for drive expression than as distinct goals, the role of objects is complex because structural theory emphasizes the control of drive expression. The drives are always evaluated in a context of their appropriateness. Thus satisfaction of the drive is tied to a standard of correctness. The ascendancy of ego psychology is notable in this regard because it vests the ego with rationality and provides for control of the irrational. Affects are important, but not as important as cognitive processes that are vital to the organizing ego functions of synthesis, integration, competence, and mastery.

Given the importance of control, how then is this a theory of separation that implies a major interest in individuality? Because it is a theory primarily about the individual mind, with a focus on ordering the expressions of the individual so that they have a logic. There is a search for meaning, and a shaping of the meaning to meet the expectations of reality. Of course the mind is not merely to be acted upon, or shaped, but can be an agent of action as well. However, its latitude is limited because reality is the ultimate arbiter, that which is, rather than a continual subjective shifting creation. On this basis then subjectivity must be subordinated to objectivity and the instinctual beast must be tamed. To see life any other way is to see it through the lens of pathology.

Narcissism is implicated in this view in a number of different ways. Pathological narcissism appears when there are failures in separation, when connections persist beyond developmental timetables, when there is a failure to differentiate and boundaries are blurred. Narcissism is seen as being in opposition to object choice in the same vein that subjectivity is contrasted with objectivity. At the same time, healthy narcissism is vested in self-esteem, in the satisfaction derived from structural integration, in the success of turning the toddler's joy at discovering the world into the adult's feelings of success at mastering life's frustrations, and basically in continuing reality adaptation. The task of the individual mind is to learn to see the world realistically and act accordingly, and the ego is the metaphorical cognitive-affective agent for such processing.

Analysis then operates as a method for the corrections of subjective distortion. The role of the analyst is to be objective, which assumes that the analyst's subjectivity has been objectified by personal analysis to the point that countertransferences can be detected and resolved. Thus, although an analysis involves two people, the patient's subjectivity is the focus while the analyst's subjectivity is thought to be reducible. Reality and objectivity are the patient's goals, and the analyst is the interpreter who is supposed to have already achieved these goals to at least the extent of becoming an accurate interpreter of the patient's subjectivity.

Another reason for the initial elevation of separation over connection was the belief in a lack of differentiation at birth and in early development that was seen as contrasting with the ultimate fate of adults to have separate identities. Because differentiation appeared to be initially missing and connection initially present, the need seemed clear. People were destined to differentiate, to form self-and-object-representations that in a variety of ways lessened connection. The latter posed the threat of a regression to symbiosis, or autism, both often equated with primary narcissism and objectlessness or objects as self-extensions, basically psychic body parts.

Another complication is that in the emphasis on separation and individuation, subjectivity is subordinated rather than cultivated as an organizing principle. The analyst learns to sift through subjectivity and arrive at objectivity, and in analysis, essentially educate patients to do the same. Cast in roles of teacher and student, the subjectivities of the analyst and the patient are less than vibrant in the analytic process.

204   Narcissism and the Relational World

Although the analyst knows so many of the patient's subjectivities, the patient appears primarily as an object. The patient does not know the analyst's subjectivities directly, and in fact the analyst often works to keep them hidden, so the analyst is also objectified. Furthermore, while they interact, the emphasis is on the analysis of distortions embodied in the transference and viewed as the window to the real source of trouble, the repression of the trauma of early relationships that disrupted drive and structural development. Intersubjectivity is blocked from consideration by the analytic structure, again limiting the conceptual range of narcissism.

Sugarman and Wilson (1995) note changes in technique that have occurred in structural approaches. There has been an expansion in the role of the analyst in transference relations, although the patient's predispositions to perceive the analyst in specific ways are still considered the major determinant of transference. The aim remains more the development of a transference neurosis than a "real" dyadic relationship. As such, separation is more the goal than connection. Also, resistance and defense, while gaining in adaptive power, retain their ties to the patient's preexisting psychic conflict rather than being patient-therapist reconstructions. The patient-therapist interaction is valued more as an experience in itself, but insight remains the major vehicle for change. This insight leads more in the direction of individuation than toward connection. Narcissism is inferred as a significant part of the patient's perceptions in the transference, particularly the part of transference that is relatively immune to the reality of the dyadic interaction.

The concept of drives as biological, motivational concepts also appears to have shifted so that motivation goes beyond drives to include relations (Sugarman, 1995), and the drives are seen as less biological. For example, Bachant, Lynch, and Richards (1995a) emphasize wishes and fantasies when describing drives, rather than tension reduction. Drives are still viewed as basic forces of motivation, but are not seen as the only determinants of behavior. Drives are depicted as one dimension of the dynamic unconscious, namely fears and wishes, but these unconscious fantasies are considered to be shaped by relationships, as well as other factors (Bachant, Lynch, & Richards, 1995b). These unconscious fantasies are of major significance to both mental and bodily functioning because they provide an interpretive viewpoint for sensory data as well as decision making. This is a narcissism of interaction, but again more one of separation than connection, because it emphasizes the development of the individual mind.

A balance seems to be suggested between biological and psychological aspects of drives. For example, Bachant et al. state, "The contemporary understanding of drive stresses the fundamental motivational significance of the individual's unique history as expressed in a dynamic unconscious that is structured by an integration of biopsychosocial determinants" (1995b, p. 568).

This makes it clear that drive is not limited to energy discharge, illustrating an awareness of the complexity of motivation, and the importance of mental representation, with a deemphasis on bodily processes. However, contemporary structural theory also seeks to retain the significance of the body, particularly in terms of not ceding too much ground to the motivational power of relations with others. Thus, Bachant et al. (1995b) point out the relationship to the body, which is personal, the influence of the body as both mediator and organizer of affective experience, and the relative motivational independence of bodily experience.

Contemporary structural theorists also tend to make the point that they do not devalue the motivational power of a relational matrix. However, even if drive theory has been turned into structural theory that wishes to be differentiated from relational theory other than on the basis of the superordinate status of instinctual, primitive drives and their derivatives, structural theory has stayed with a focus on individual development and the growth of the individual mind. This is a matter of emphasis and does include giving considerable motivational power to object relationships. In the long run these relationships, through the medium of identification, become socializing and thereby controlling influences on the drives. In that sense, the superordinate motivation could well be viewed as drive control through the medium of object relations, with its indentificatory models, as contrasted with drive gratification. This view is apparent in the idea of drive neutralization (Hartmann, 1950), and in the suggestion by Brenner (1993) that behavior is formed through the influences of drive derivatives, affects, defenses and the superego. Thus growth through separation and the development of individual identities ends up with connection in the form of socialization at the very least as part of a necessary adaptive process. The distinction between structural and relational theories actually resides in the reason for an ultimate integration of biopsychosocial factors. In structural theory this integration is an evolutionary, biological necessity rather than a desire for connection.

All the motivational components of an unbridled narcissism are present, namely the search for gratification, the focus on individuality, and the pleasure principle, but ultimately as Lasky notes, there are "the regulatory principles of mental functioning" (1993, p.25). Because connection is not sought out primarily for its own sake, but more as a means to an end, then separation remains as an unfulfilled wish that periodically may seek satisfaction and requires defensive adaptations. Subjectivity is on the one-hand highly valued as a motivational component, yet devalued due to being a frequent source of maladaptation via personally inappropriate attempts at drive gratification. Objectivity is more the goal, and even if viewed as a consensus of sufficient subjectivities, there is at best room for relative uniqueness, which it could be argued, is the path of least subjectivity. Although connections throughout the life span are of great utility, the ability to take care of the self has greater value than to be taken care of by others, and the ability to take care of others is to be balanced by the establishment of self-sustenance in order to avoid a masochistic adaptation. This emphasis on separation highlights a major task for narcissism, namely the development of mechanisms for soothing the self, mechanisms that can both use objects and be of use to objects, all aimed at establishing an ongoing potential for self-sufficiency. The personal perspective is developed with conscious and unconscious imperatives for conflict resolution amidst the metaphorical structures that are created to represent desires and capacities.

What desires and what capacities are offered in separation theory? Libido and aggression in their myriad, often fused forms describe the desires, whereas the capacities are depicted particularly as ego functions. However, the emphasis need not be on what resides where, or even on the existence of structures, but on the power of desire and the ability of the person to organize the expression of desire. Psychic energy was a useful concept in this regard, but its literal quantification was a burden and it has fallen out of favor. Perhaps the affects have become its replacement, in essence the feelings for and about life that express an energic state. These feelings are also intertwined with cognition, so that the affect is usually expressed in a conceptual, symbolized manner, as in the statement, "I am angry." Whether arising swiftly with little apparent thought, or expressed after deliberation, the statement represents the organization of desire and involves both the desire and the capacities to express the desire.

The major legacy of structural theory that is there for narcissism is the centrality of desire, which is even more powerful if the instinctual, biological nature of desire is indeed insisted upon as a major motivational force. The structural apparatus, ego and superego especially, depict the context of control, so desire becomes socialized as adaptation. However, separation is considered more inherent to desire than connection, which is more of an instrument than the goal. Narcissism embodies self-sufficiency, the overcoming of deficits and the resolution of conflicts through relationships, but not inherently for the sake of relationships. Healthy narcissism is successful separation-individuation, whereas pathological narcissism reflects distorted connectedness, be it isolation or fusion.

Of course structural theory does not ignore either the effects or value of connections with others. It also keeps subjectivity within the boundaries of objectivity, as well as allowing for the influence of the personal on reality so that the latter is not eternally fixed. However, even if the dual-instinct concept is not considered as life and death, the individual does traverse a course from connection to separation. Thus structural theory, even if drives are conceptualized more as wishes and fears than biologically-based instincts, is a theory of transitional relations that in their demands often foster conflict and ultimately require dissolution. Narcissism becomes the negotiation of passages. This is particularly well illustrated in the process of analysis itself where the transference neurosis is developed and in turn dissolved; connection made, separation is to follow.

The process does aim at a release of pathological connections so that there is indeed room for better connections. Nonetheless, in a form that parallels the relationship with the analyst but has more specific latitude, healthier connections are balanced to emphasize individuation, particularly in the form of the potential for self-sufficiency that makes bearable the inevitable loss of relations. The dominant ultimate relationship is the relationship to the self, and structural analytic technique that stresses transference formation and interpretation, highlights self-relationships.

Thus both classical drive theory and its current revision, contemporary structural theory, provide us with an understanding of one significant aspect of narcissism, namely separation as the major component of drive expression. This is carried out within a context of conflict, defense control, and adaptive resolution. Connection is part of the separation-individuation process, rather than being an equal partner in the drive motivation. Although object relations have grown in importance in structural theory it is logically consistent with the theory that they be subordinated to the organization of structure designed to resolve conflict and establish psychic equilibrium. In so doing, separation is emphasized as a key ingredient of narcissism.

Connection

Relational theory has provided a reevaluation of connection as an enabling process and transformed connection into a basic human desire. The result is a reversal of structural theory so that now separations are way-stations to the sought-after destinations of connection. As a result differentiation is an aspect of interaction with others and occurs within a relational context that furthers the goal of connection. Identity becomes more an issue of being part of an interactive matrix than of being distinct from others.

Of course, just as with structural theory, there are specific variations within relational theory. In developing an integration for relational theory, Mitchell (1988) notes the three approaches of relational by design, by intent, and by implication. Also, some relational theorists view the individual as relatively undifferentiated at birth, similar to structural theory, whereas others see the infant as relatively differentiated. However, relational theory has a central theme of connection. Differentiation itself becomes a way to recognize the existence of others outside of the self and in turn develop connections. The psychology of the interpersonal field now becomes of greater interest than the psychology of the individual mind. The person is seen as innately a social being, predisposed to interact with others, with experience arising and accumulating from these interactions. These social relations are viewed as basic biological motivations, akin to the drives of structural theory, but not identical. Thus the body is not left behind, but libido and aggression are operating as physiological responses that function within a relational field, and derive their meaning from these relations. Libido and aggression tend not to be viewed as instincts or as primary motivators, but as modes of relatedness. Just as structural theory takes notice of the role of relationships but retains a drive emphasis, so relational theory includes libido and aggression as involved in motivation, but emphasizes their relational base.

Narcissism as a cathexis of the self, or as a "cathexis" of anything, does not fit comfortably with relational theory, but the idea of narcissism as a personal perspective seems quite appropriate. In this vein narcissism is a subjective view of interaction, a strategy for engagement, whose health or pathology rests upon the successful development of connections with others. Pathological narcissism is perhaps most apparent in separation and isolation, although self-serving connections also provide opportunities for narcissistic distortion. There is an evaluative element to connectedness, which instead of evoking the objective reality of structural theory, uses the standard of mutual satisfaction for subject and object. The norm is cooperation, measured in degrees of intersubjectivity, with the shadow of others providing the surround for the life of the individual.

The deemphasis of separation unfortunately at times leads to using narcissism as an overall description of antagonism to object relations, a problem also noted in structural theory, although for different reasons. Narcissism represents in both relational and structural theory an organizational perspective. In relational theory the observation of interaction, the recognition of differentiation, and the apparent need for attachment, are all seen as signs of the supremacy of attachment, which in turn is reflective of self-organization as connection.

The presence and motivating power of interaction, as well as the motivation for interaction (Bowlby, 1969; Lichtenberg, 1983) are not so much in dispute as are the reasons for connection. For example, in relational theory interaction is often viewed as pleasurable in itself, supporting the idea of interactive narcissism. This line of thought is helpful in validating the idea of early differentiation and therefore recognition of objects outside of the self, but it is not convincing in terms of establishing a motivational force that has to be distinct from what is contained in the libidinal and aggressive drives. In essence the properties of interaction that make it sought after will not appear sufficiently distinct from pleasure seeking unless pleasure is redefined and thereby divided into a number of specific categories. On that basis "contact pleasure" or "interaction gratification" should have meanings and values that are distinct from libidinal or aggressive pleasures. However, it is not clear that such pleasures are so distinct, nor is it clear that being programmed to interact is a major motivational force that is superordinate to libido and aggression. Being social by design could be seen as primarily a description of drive control, a basic feature of structural theory. To get beyond such a view it is necessary to posit something special, basic, and encompassing about socialization, and to make libido and aggression means for socialization rather than primary goals.

The question is, does viewing the infant as inherently social essentially subordinate the drives? Not necessarily, because the drives as depicted in contemporary structural theory are redesigned to develop as a relational field while keeping intact their instinctual roots. Instead inherent socialization would make the experience of relating the most satisfactory form of drive expression. Or, if one wishes to delete the concept of drive, then interactional experiences would be viewed as the major sources of human need satisfaction, although not the only sources.

However, even if it were to be argued that all human needs are primarily relational, thereby viewing narcissism as a relational perspective, there still remains the question of what is the fundamental reason for relations being satisfying. Contemporary structural theory is both a recognition of the limitations of drive-discharge motivation, and a reaction to it, but certainly a different reaction than relational theory. The latter takes the view that observational data support the significant presence of human interaction from birth, and imply the predisposition for such interaction, as well as suggesting that this interaction provides many satisfactions. However, that is not equivalent to demonstrating that there is an inherent goal of interaction that would account for preadapted potentials.

Actually, relational theory often goes beyond a socialization-by-nature view to suggest one or more reasons for social interaction that explain the value of relationships. Thus Fairbairn (1952) hypothesizes that the major human motivation is seeking relationships because they provide the satisfaction of contact, which is differentiated from pleasure. Thus some sought-after relationships can be painful, others can bring pleasure, but the contact is a needed satisfaction. In this view narcissism has a major theme of considering contact as an organizing perspective.

Of course it can be argued that pain and pleasure are not necessarily opposites, that sometimes the pleasure is the pain, but in this differentiation pleasure and pain are narrowly defined to distinguish the relational motivation from structural drive motivation. The desire for relatedness continues to be viewed as innate, but with greater elaboration of the reasons for such a given, and learning is used to account for different styles of connectedness. The elaboration suggests a basic motive, or basic motives, however, that would underlie the desire for relationships.

For example, establishing and maintaining a sense of self may appear as the dominant motivation, but this identity is essentially dependent on the establishment of relationships. Thus what appears as a foundation motive, namely identity for the sake of organization, is proposed as the reason for relatedness which is at the same time essential to establishing identity. Actually this view fits with the drive management focus of structural theory where the ego would serve as an organizing metaphor and relations are needed for the development of the ego, but the emphasis is not on the relations. In relational theory, relations are not only essential links to identity or organization, or even structural development, but all these concepts are in themselves relational.

It does seem that structural and relational theories are potentially overlapping, depending on how their components are interpreted. In all of the relational models, even if it were to be argued that connectedness is the nature of humanity, the reason for that nature bears consideration. In that consideration the idea that people derive pleasure from relating, that it has adaptive value, that it organizes, stabilizes, and provides an identity, all sound akin to the postulates of structural theory.

Mitchell (1988) has examined the possibilities for model mixing, namely that the relational model was and is implicit in drive theory, or that while relational theory is distinct, it is compatible with structural theory and a logical extension of it, or finally that the models do not mix conceptually. He supports the last alternative and considers relational theory the best approach, which of course would be disputed by structural theorists as well as theorists seeking an integration of the theories. Clearly this is a controversial issue which lacks a definitive answer.

Jordan et al. (1991) also opt for a strong relational approach that while focused on women's development, does not have to be gendered. The model involves a switch from separation-individuation to relationship-differentiation. Differentiation in this model is redefined as a "dynamic process that encompasses increasing levels of complexity, structure, and articulation within the context of human bonds and attachments" (p. 36). This is a "self-in-relation" model that emphasizes connections based on feeling states and identification that result in a *mutual reciprocity*. The motivation for the mutuality appears to be a pleasure in relatedness. This is defined as "the ability to identify with the other, the sense of connectedness through feeling states, and the *activation* and *energizing*...involving the awareness of the needs and/or 'reality' of another person as well as one's own" (p. 37).

Connection is not considered the only developmental line, with other possibilities acknowledged such as agency and competence, but relational needs are viewed as primary. Thus identity exists in relation to others and the pleasure of connection is not equivalent to the libidinal pleasure of structural theory. The self is seen as beginning with an interest in others which gains expression in connection and the ability to empathize. There is an expectation of mutuality in which shared experience furthers the development of both the self and others. Interaction is viewed as essential for growth, and interaction is equated with mutual sensitivity and responsibility. This relational model casts narcissism in the perspective of mutual intersubjectivity. The individual is motivated to organize the self not only in relational terms, but in relational terms that stress the inner experience of others on a basis that is equivalent to an interest in one's own inner world. Thus, intrinsic pleasure is derived from the mutuality, the intersubjectivity of relationships which in turn are the best form of connectedness.

It is not clear, however, why this would come about. The theory asserts that personal growth will be maximized by feeling connected, yet separation theory asserts the opposite, emphasizing the pleasures of competition and individuation. Certainly there are attractions in mutuality, but neither the presence of intersubjectivity nor the gratification of mutual connections are sufficient to provide connection with a superordinate status. The movement from subjectivity to intersubjectivity remains a mysterious process in terms of its motivation, an issue that appears also in self-psychology in terms of attempting to explain why the movement occurs from using a selfobject to being a selfobject for another person. The movement indeed occurs, and intersubjectivity is a recognizable interactive state with is own satisfaction for the participants, but that is not equivalent to intrinsic motivation.

Mitchell (1988) suggests viewing relational theory as encompassing rather than discretely motivational. A social nature is posited, but with many options for expression of connection, all of which provide motivational possibilities, and some of these will dominate in each individual. Some examples cited are security, dependency, mutual knowing, and pleasure. This view, however, does not alter the impression that relational theory and structural theory encompass each other with the main distinctions residing in what are emphasized as the basic units of study.

For narcissism the personal perspective in relational theory has to include relations with others. Pathological narcissism would involve distorted interpersonal relations and alienation, and any perspective that stressed separation over connection would reflect a narcissistic disturbance. Thus in the area of relations the narcissism of structural and relational theory could differ, with the structural theory emphasizing individuation in contrast to the interrelatedness of relational theory. However, if structural and relational theories are viewed as potentially complementary, then narcissism expands beyond contrasting views of what is healthy to provide insights into integrating self and relational expression. The self develops in a relational context, but it is insufficient to position identity as a relational concept, or to view the individual as striving to be in relationships. There is an issue of the separate self that merits attention, and narcissism has as its unending task the taking apart and putting together of separate and connected states of being, a task that is actually depicted quite well in the concept of mutuality.

Jordan et al. (1991) describe mutuality as mutual intersubjectivity. The components of this model are interest in, awareness of, and response to the subjectivity of the other; self-disclosure; personal need acknowledgment without manipulation to gain gratification; valuing the growth of the other; and establishing interactions where both parties are open to change. Although the motivations for this type of mutuality are partially learned, there is thought to be an intrinsic value to such interaction. This model is in contrast to separation and is formed on the evidence for early capacities for relating and an early development of the sense of self that is an *interpersonal identity*. Thus the self is primarily, if not exclusively, interactive. There is an ongoing awareness of being distinct, a self-integrity, but it is in the context of being connected to others. In fact, the differences between the self and others are established through interaction.

This version of mutuality requires that the narcissistic perspective be intersubjective on an ongoing basis. The "natural tendency" in this model is to connect, so that the task of narcissism is weighted in the direction of reconciling and integrating senses of separateness with the prevailing sense of connection. The idea of an intrinsic motivation to connect, the many adaptive advantages of connection, and the idealism of an intersubjectivity are all quite appealing, but they are no more convincing than separation theory. Giving superordinate status to either view seems to essentially be a narcissistic decision, namely a personal preference for varying degrees of separation and connection.

Aron (1996) notes that there are different kinds of mutuality. For example, mutuality of recognition emphasizes the ability of people to acknowledge each other as separate subjects. Mutuality of regulation considers reciprocal control in relationships. The common thread for all types of mutuality, however, is a joint endeavor. The common thread for all types of narcissism is a personal perspective, but a perspective that is both autonomous and connected to others.

Can that be? In contemporary relational theory separation is a dynamic concept, so that a personal perspective exists as an integral part of connection. The same view can be found in contemporary structural theory, except that the primacy of the personal perspective is emphasized so that relations exist within the capacities of individuality. Both views accept the idea of relational coconstructions, as well as coconstructions of individuality, but shift the primary formative force. Mutuality is present throughout, but expressed in different ways. For example, the dichotomy of subject-object is more apparent in the structural approach. Relational-perspectivism (Aron, 1996) provides an awareness of asymmetrical coparticipation, whereas mutual empathy (Jordan et al., 1991) requires an exceptional intersubjectivity.

Actually, none of this is the best fit for understanding narcissism. Basically, separation theory is too separate, and connection theory is too connected. Narcissism as a personal perspective reflects greater fluidity in which there are indeed many absolute, radical moments of both separation and connection that are not to be viewed as pathological. Thus in considering the influence of connection on narcissism, it is not acceptable to always view identity as relational, although identity certainly does appear to develop more within a relational context than outside of it. That however, does not mean that identity rests on the recognition of the other as subject and/or object, or that the self has to differentiate to survive. Certainly recognition and differentiation occur, and frequently, but at the same time, the self will stand alone and will step outside of others in the creation and preservation of an active inner life. There are times of "just being" and there are times of "being-in-relation," as well as those "in-between" states that are basically everyday, healthy experiences.

Commentary
Thus instead of coming down on either side, namely structural or relational, which have been symbolized in separation and connection, the view is to favor attempting integrations that will take into account both the polarized and the complementary aspects of separation and connection. This reflects searching for a solution that illuminates the substantial centrality of narcissism. It is intriguing that the emphasis on separation found in structural theory gives way to the rule of objectivity, apparently conceding there is danger in the triumph of the individual mind. Socialization prevails out of necessity however, rather than pleasure. In that vein, separation theory is insufficiently individualized, thereby not giving enough room for healthy narcissism.

At the same time the emphasis on connection found in relational theory begins with differentiation as a way to recognize the self and others. Subjectivity is thus made apparent, but is ultimately shaded in the direction of paying marked attention to the subjectivity of others and thereby emphasizing connection. Socialization is emphasized now as the pleasurable goal. From that point of view, connection theory is not subjective enough to provide sufficient space for healthy narcissism. Both approaches veer in the direction of making narcissism a term primarily for pathological subjective enactments, which in turn inaccurately restricts the concept of narcissism. Also, although separation theory has shed considerable light on narcissism in terms of understanding the workings of the individual mind, its emphasis on objectivity is a problem for conceptualizing narcissism. Connection theory has made major contributions to understanding narcissism in its delineation of the role of subjectivity in relations, but the ultimate goal is relatedness and that too is a problem for depicting narcissism. Of course, neither of these models appear consistently in such categorical forms as just described, but it is fair to say that neither supports the motivational primacy of an individual perspective. Structural theory limits narcissism in service of various types of social and moral adaptation, and connection theory emphasizes the social nature of the self, the relational individual. As a result what is available does not appear to address sufficiently what is a major concern as well as being a basic asset in the concept of narcissism, namely the motivational power of subjectivity. In that regard, it appears that although concepts such as coconstruction certainly illustrate subjective roles as motivational, still the "co" part is a restriction on subjectivity. However, Aron (1996) convincingly illustrates the inevitability of subjectivity for the analyst in the clinical situation, leaving room for the possibility that at times what may pass as a coconstruction is two separate personal constructions that work out to be positive, satisfactory activities for the analyst and the patient.

Granted that when two constructions take place in the presence of two interacting people, it would appear that there is a coconstruction, even if one person is silent, or inattentive, or psychically somewhere else for the entire session, because the assumption is that the two people are reacting to each other. However, what if they are not? The very definition of a therapy session would say that they are, and it is appropriate to call the analyst and patient "interacting people" because one knows there is always some kind of interaction during the session. At the same time, there can be many moments of noninteraction, where both members of the dyad are not having anything to do with each other. For example, the patient stops speaking to the analyst although the patient keeps talking and the analyst stops listening to the patient although the analyst keeps listening. These moments could occur at the same time for analyst and patient, or different times, and they could go unnoticed by either patient or analyst. It is quite possible that neither therapists or patients are that attuned to each other that such dissociative states are always noticed, nor is it inevitable that these states are always caused by the interaction in the dyad.

It is understood of course that analysts are supposed to pay attention to patients, and patients are in therapy to get something from a situation that includes their therapists, so interaction and coconstruction are to be expected and are powerful therapeutic tools. It is also known that authoritative interpretation, as well as strong resistances, are often conconstructed, and that there will be empathic misattunements as well as countertransference enactments. All in all, the dissociative subjective state, dissociative in that at least one person is now out of the interaction, looks like an obstacle to therapeutic progress, and is generally thought of as a reactive state that will need to be altered.

However, that may not always be the case. For example, consider an instance in which the analyst falls asleep during the session, and awakens before the session ends without the patient having an apparent awareness that the analyst was asleep. The use of the modifier, "apparent," is because of course at some level of consciousness the patient may sense the analyst's lack of participation, but it is also possible that such is not the case. In such an instance the conconstruction is absent from the analyst's point of view because the analyst was not there. Now add to this situation that the dissociative state of sleep is not caused by the analyst's reaction to the patient, but by fatigue. Similar situations could be developed for temporary distractions, and dissociative states on the part of patients could also occur that are not reactive to the analyst or the analytic situation.

Let us now take this issue a step further and conjecture that some type of nonreactive separateness occurs often in analytic sessions because both members of the dyad have the same needs in and out of sessions, namely to both separate and connect, that is a subjective organizing activity. The need to be separate is at times motivated by the current situation of the person, including either the situation itself or associations to it. These are reactive separations, but there are also nonreactive separations motivated by states of mind that are dominant at that time. Sometimes interaction dominates, but other times isolation prevails, regardless of the interaction and dissociated from it.

Aron (1996) comments on a contrasting set of needs within individuals, namely to know the other and be known by the other as opposed to not knowing the other and being left alone. These needs are cast in relational terms and in the models depicted by Winnicott (1965) and Rank (1945). In turn the analytic situation is pictured as an ongoing conflictual interaction between these needs in the patient and in the analyst, where both revealing and concealing are inevitable. One can agree with this, but can also see it as commonplace that the analytic situation contains ongoing intrapersonal phases as well that coexist with the interpersonal, but can be discrete from it as well as connected. As a result it is possible to interpret both Winnicott and Rank somewhat differently. Their models can be seen as relational, yet give an emphasis to the self-communication described by Winnicott (1965) as something different from interactive relational communication. Instead it represents a need to continually have a personal perspective that is sometimes referenced to others, either by connection or separation, disclosure or concealment, but at other times is referenced only to the feelings and ideas of the individual doing and thinking. In a similar vein Rank's autonomy of the self can represent a movement away from others, but it can also be viewed as a periodic reorganizing activity that is internally focused for its own sake. This is not designed as an avoidance of

218 Narcissism and the Relational World

interaction, but as a self-interaction that has the same subject and object, and coexists with interaction in fluctuations of focus from subjectivity to being interpersonal to being subjective. This is a process that is sometimes a dialogue, and in that sense dialectical in relation to an other, and at other times a monologue, dialectical in a within-the-self context and different from reactions to or from others.

Intersubjectivity is an illustration of the issues involved in formulating the personal perspective of narcissism in the context of connection. Jordan et al. (1991) describe intersubjectivity as an example of "subject relations" in which the other person is experienced as a subject, and relationships and identity have a synchronous movement. In the model, there is no separate self, but a self within relationships. There are ongoing desires for connection, increasing capacities for mutual empathy, and desires to protect and nurture relationships. Even self-empathy is seen in a relational matrix. The individual is motivated to relate, and furthermore to relate in an empathic intersubjectivity. The separating self is equated with the separate self and seen as reactive to the complexities or difficulties of relating. This is in contrast to the view that there are intrapersonal and interpersonal selves, and that a personal perspective is the dominant organizing force. In that view the self often steps outside of relations, as well as being in them, for reasons that sometimes have to do with interpersonal relations, but at other times are intrapersonal. The formation of the self happens in a relational environment, but this does not mean that the motivation is necessarily relational. It may be that self-development is motivated by organizing principles that meet a variety of personal needs, such as stability, agency, coherence, and community. The basic motivation is need satisfaction that is registered by the self in affective terms. A personal perspective, narcissism, is the decision maker as to need-satisfying behavior. On this basis, a person is not motivated to connect, or to separate, for the sake of either connection or separation, but because these activities are conceptualized as personally satisfying. Aron (1996) takes note of this aspect of narcissism when he describes an interplay between two dimensions of the self, namely a separate sense of subjectivity, and the self as an object, as well as the other as both subject and object. The development of these aspects of the self, really the multiplicity of identity, is congruent with the concept of narcissism, but even the asymmetrical mutuality that is suggested by Aron contains a relational basis that as a motivational force could be dissonant with narcissism as an organizing perspective.

Benjamin (1995a) emphasizes the tension that exists in the maintenance of intersubjectivity. Each individual is motivated by the pleasures of mutuality and sharing, yet there is an awareness of differences that frequently results in what could be described as a complimentary mutuality. These relationships are inevitably conflictual, marked by disturbances and subsequent separation. Mutual recognition appears as a developmental task and an accomplishment, but with the understanding that there will be continual imbalance between subjectivity and intersubjectivity. Benjamin appears to view both experiences as significantly motivating self development without necessarily giving one precedence over the other, although the intrapsychic subjective self seems to remain essentially a relational self, motivated into existence to relate to the other as object and subject. Thus in connection theory the individual standing alone is a separated individual reacting to a relational matrix in some fashion and motivated by relational constructs. This is of course in contrast to the individuating force that underlies separation theory, but separation is the result of differentiation, so that the individual has again become distinctive in a reactive fashion. Although different from connection theory, separation theory is then also relational, and self development as a function of differentiation is relational regardless of adherence to separation or connection theory.

However, these conclusions are not equivalent to conceptualizing motivation as primarily relational because the development of relations may well be for satisfactions other than relating. The movement from the primacy of separation to the primacy of connection has provided for a fuller understanding of the role of relations in the development of the self, and clearly made narcissism a more complex construct. The introduction of intersubjectivity highlights continual subject-object interactions that also require a deeper understanding of narcissism as a subjective experience. Neither separation theory nor connection theory, however, would give narcissism the emphasis or force that it appears to have. The primary motivational force is instead conceptualized as constructive self development in which the self is drawn to whatever it perceives provides the greatest satisfaction for its multiple needs. Separation and connection are certainly among these needs, but they are an overlap to what will be considered personal satisfaction. One separates and connects to make the self feel good, and it is the individual person who decides what it means to "feel good."

Self-psychology as originally formulated (Kohut, 1971a) required a partial differentiation from selfobjects and a significant takeover of their functions, but they were never completely relinquished. In addition, selfobjects appeared to be objects serving the needs of a subject, so that empathy flowed from the selfobjects to the subject, as contrasted with mutual empathy. So it was a theory of connection in that the ultimate goal was not separation, but more the retention of varying degrees of connection. However, the connection appeared to fall short of an authentic intersubjectivity. The motivation for the person to become a selfobject is somewhat unclear, but it is being addressed in contemporary self-psychology through the elaboration of a potential range of selfobject functions (Bacal, 1990). There is potential adaptive value in being a selfobject in that it provides the reward of facilitating the progression of generations of developmental cycles, e.g., it is good parenting. The idea of connection rather than separation appears dominant because autonomy is relative, part of a cohesive self that always includes the presence of selfobjects. Selfobjects are used to designate functions that contribute to a cohesive self, or more precisely, the subjective experience of such functions. This takes us back to narcissism, a personal perspective on what best serves the self. These experiences often take place in what Stolorow views as an intersubjective field where two subjectivities interact, but from an internal observational position (Stolorow, Brandchaft, & Atwood, 1987). The narcissitic need for a cohesive self supports the value of selfobject functions such as empathy and wisdom that are significant aspects of connection and intersubjectivity.

The inevitability of conflict and ambivalence in relationships described by Greenberg (1991) is similar to the tension in relating that has been described by both Benjamin (1995a) and Aron (1996), although these two authors are more definite about the goal of conflict resolution being connection. However, their view of connection does take into account an ongoing separation-connection lifetime struggle. Greenberg comes closer to the view of a *separateness*, rather than separation, that is involved in narcissism, in his belief in a nondefensive and nonresistive separation, although he does describe it as "nonrelatedness." Instead, individuals could be considered as existing within themselves both when they are alone and when they are with others. Thus there is always an intrapersonal dialogue about the most beneficial personal perspective. This idea is reflected in Benjamin's view of the intrapsychic and

Greenberg's view of a type of conflict that is not connected to others, although these authors do not link their views to narcissism.

The separation-connection issue is also demonstrated in regard to technique, particularly in regard to the concept of disclosure by the analyst, a revelation of subjectivity that is often viewed as an expression of some type of narcissism. Aron (1996) believes that an analysis is a coconstruction, that self-disclosure of some sort is inevitable, and that purposeful self-disclosure can be useful, but he believes its value depends on both the individual patient and the individual analyst. In his view it is an option, neither required nor prohibited, but worked out within the therapeutic situation. This could mean that deliberate self-disclosure is then a matter of the analyst's personal judgment, which can be translated into the analyst making use of a personal perspective.

Greenberg (1991) approaches the issue differently, emphasizing the value of a neutral stance, but seeing neutrality as a therapeutic form. He states, "The neutral analyst occupies a position that maintains an optimal tension between the patient's tendency to see him as a dangerous object and the capacity to experience him as a safe one" (p. 217). There is a coconstruction in this view also because the patient provides the initial material for the analyst's intervention, as well as the feedback as to the evaluation of what is "optimal." At the same time, it is the analyst who is making the judgment as to what constitutes a neutral position. Thus it seems that neutrality is also a reflection of a personal perspective. Ultimately the analyst's narcissism sets the tone for the analysis.

Friedman (1997) approaches the issue of technique with still another perspective. He suggest two essentials, an adversarial attitude and a search for objective truth. The adversarialness is essentially a skepticism about what the patient presents, a deconstruction of the patient's meanings and view, with the aim of arriving at the truth, which of course assumes that there is an objective truth. There is a coconstruction here, but it is in service of a mutual task that emphasizes the patient's subjectivity more than the analyst's. This implies more of a separation emphasis than a connection one, because the analytic relationship remains relatively depersonalized with interpretation aimed continually at objectivity. An objective interpretation tries to indicate that it is "just how it is," as compared with "this is my opinion," but the former is still the creation of the person making the interpretation. Thus, the comparison between subjective and objective interpretations rest on the degree of the interpreter's personal investment in the interpretation.

The result is at best a relative objectivity, clouded even further by the probabilities of unconscious subjectivities in interpretation.

Nonlinear Lines

The development of psychoanalytic theory and practice from an emphasis on separation to an emphasis on connection has not been linear and neat, but jagged and messy. Nonetheless psychoanalytic work has become more relationally oriented, whether motives such as drives are used as underpinning for relations, or attachment itself is considered a basic motive. A major result of this relational tilt is the increased recognition of the role of the analyst's subjectivity, which is another way of saying that narcissism is having a rebirth (although the term itself is not so frequently employed). Furthermore, the analyst's subjectivity is not derided as a countertransferential force in need of a speedy resolution once it is noticed, but the value of subjectivity is being explored as a therapeutic force. Thus the analyst no longer struggles to be neutral in the way the concept was originally proposed, because this is a struggle the analyst is bound to lose (Renik, 1996). Instead the analyst accepts narcissism and attempts to use it constructively.

The question is, what is constructive? The answer to this is complicated by the fact that the evolution of psychoanalysis has changed the therapeutic tasks. They have multiplied, although the burden is usually eased by picking a set of goals that cluster around the analyst's personal vision of mental health. Analysts try to influence their patients to focus on certain problems, to look at these problems in particular ways, and to resolve the problems in a certain manner. Intriguingly, one of these ways is to get patients to make up their own minds, to follow their narcissism, and in that sense, to suspend the part of the analyst's influence that is incongruent with what the patient considers the best personal course of action. That suspension is the co-construction aspect of connection theory, which also includes patients influencing the analyst in specific ways.

However, it is as Aron (1996) notes, an asymmetrical mutuality. In dispute are two related issues at the heart of analysis, authority and transference. If the establishment of transference is considered essential by the analyst, then expressions of subjectivity that emphasize self-disclosure are likely to slant the transference, or to reduce it, because the space for projected fantasies has been narrowed. Let us grant here that some patients are persistent about their transferences, and relatively impervious to contrary evidence. Nonetheless, if the thrust of the analysis is to provide as much room as possible for the patient's fantasies about the analyst, then analytic anonymity helps. It also reduces the degree of analyst-influence that is known to the analyst. There may never be a blank screen, nor will analysts ever operate equidistant from id, ego, and superego, but the analyst has and uses options about the self that can limit or expand transference. What is the best path? Each analyst, in process and/or in advance, makes a personal decision, and knows, but the knowing has gotten more difficult, with so many choices, all open to challenge.

> What is it that a psychoanalyst wishes to do? Is the principal task of an analyst to create an environment in which the patient will feel secure? Or is it to assist the patient to become able to analyze him or herself? Or to repair defects in the patient's ego functioning? Does an analyst wish mainly to improve the patient's sense of self? Or to help the patient discover how the patient reacts to the analyst's words, tone of voice, and general behavior? Or is an analyst's chief wish to discover the nature and development of the patient's pathogenic conflicts and to convey that information to the patient? (Brenner, 1996, p.21).

What is striking about the quote from Brenner is the acknowledgment of the personal nature of the analyst's desires in the therapeutic process. Also, although Brenner is clear that for him the task of analysis is to understand and interpret a patient's conflict, how one understands and interprets again become subjective operations. However, one is not without broad guidelines, because once the analyst's task is chosen, then certain activities, such as the fostering or diminution of the transference, are likely to follow. The narcissism lies in the belief about the transference, and the particulars of carrying out the belief.

Transference reflects the authority of the analyst, with negative transference tending to depreciate it or turning it into a fearful force, but positive transference tending to reinforce it. Usually there is a role transference prior to the analysis that certainly carries into it, and the analyst is seen in the role of an authority. Postmodernism, deconstructionism, and mutuality as part of the relational tilt have a number of different views as to what to do with the patients' assumptions of analysts' authority. Friedman (1996) points out that with a few exceptions, there is an increasing skepticism about what the analyst can know, and a movement away from searching for objective truth which is replaced with mutual reflection. At the same time this is tempered by what Kernberg (1996) refers to as a functional authority in which the analyst leads in a collaborative activity.

With the emphasis on connection and mutuality in practice, reevaluations of transference and countertransference occur. The analyst's personal judgments about the utility of transference are now more the criteria for how transference is worked into a session. The same issue appears for countertransference. These once-basic features of analysis are now shifting variables. For example, a common guideline of the past was the relative anonymity of the analyst which required the patient to essentially guess what the therapist felt and thought about the patient's productions. The guess was viewed as a projection, based on past experiences with significant others. This transference was considered an essential pathway for the analyst and patient to gain an understanding of the patient that neither had, or would have, without transference. Self-disclosure by the analyst was kept to a minimum because of the potential for interfering with the transference. Although there was certainly a subjective element to both the timing and content of intervention by the analyst, the general guideline of primarily listening was a boundary for the expression of subjectivity. The fostering of transference in an environment created by the analyst to hide analytic subjectivity and to search for an objective truth that the analyst was expected to be capable of knowing as well as transmitting, given the cooperation of the patient, was the general order of the day.

Contrast this with the view that patient and analyst create transference and countertransference as a contingent process that emphasizes the encounter between two people in the present (Chodorow, 1996). There is an emphasis on unpredictability, novelty, discontinuity, and confusion (Elliot & Spezzano, 1996), and in particular, on personal meaning (Mitchell, 1993). The increased recognition of subjectivities in the analytic encounter is a demonstration of the power of narcissism as both a healthy and pathological motivational force.

The threat of pathological narcissism lies both in the exercise of authority and the abandonment of authority. The belief that the analyst either usually or even always "knows best" created the opportunity for unrecognized subjective expressions that could be exploitative, which when recognized were classified as countertransferential. Recognition was less likely in the objective model, however, because the assumed probability of the analyst's correctness was high. In the current subjective model the possibility of dialogue and corrective feedback is encouraged by the analyst, so mistakes or attempted exploitations are easier to notice and to change. Thus the authority is lessened when the analyst emphasizes connection.

At the same time, the connection model is more likely to create a sense of threatening unease for both patient and analyst because of the relative lack of a recognized authority. An emphasis on concepts each as emergent meanings and ongoing uncertainty create a tension that the analyst may be tempted to resolve by continually diminishing responsibility through relinquishing authority. In that case the pathological narcissism appears under the guise of mutuality and providing greater freedom of choice for the patient without however helping the patient to develop a position that is sufficiently secure for the patient to make better choices than were being made prior to therapy.

Thus separation and connection theories both carry their share of danger for patients, and emphasize the need for guidelines that are vested in some type of authority being held by the analyst. As analysts are more aware of the subjectivity of all their decisions, it is clear that objective truth is at best relative truth, and there are multiple possibilities, or "many truths," any one of which may prove to be effective in a particular course of therapy.

Friedman (1996) takes note of this multiplicity in his overview of a series of articles on knowledge and authority in the psychoanalytic relationship. For example, suggested approaches include focusing on the present, making some judgments openly, being receptive to different types of awareness, being more playful, and increasing mutuality. Of course, as Friedman points out, all of these reflect a belief in what works best and how to do it, namely knowledge and authority. Furthermore, all of it is subjective, and remains open to empirical testing, which in turn will be open to subjective interpretation, so, without endorsing one approach over another, notice can again be taken of the narcissistic nature of the whole enterprise.

The subjectivity of the analyst has always been recognized, but earlier thinking saw it as a feature that was much more reducible than the way it is now viewed, and also, as a characteristic that was more likely to be harmful than helpful to the analysis. This previous view was more a component of the belief that meaning was more objective for both analyst and patient than it now appears to be. The relationship within the dyad was always considered to be vital, but more limited than at present because of the focus on facilitating a transference. Thus in the movement from separation to connection many uncertainties have arisen, particularly in regard to technique, at the same time that new theoretical possibilities have been created, such as the greater level of differentiation that is present in the infant from birth. Modifications of both structural and relational theories continue to occur, and it is actually the interpretations of these theories that become the guidelines for technique. These subjective impressions are essentially theories of behavior that analysts believe are the most accurate ways to understand people. Then, based on these impressions, analysts translate them into technique, now with a marked recognition that there will be a personal flavor to both the understanding of the theory and its implementation, so that there is more variability and in turn, less uniformity, to each and every analysis. The variability is to be expected and to be used in a positive way to customize the analysis, providing a better dyadic fit than if the subjectivities of both parties were not so recognized, or if recognized, were thought of mainly as an interference.

Renik (1996) has pointed out that the analyst's activity involves communicating personal judgments. Recognizing this increases the analyst's responsibility, particularly in terms of clarifying with the patient that an intervention is at heart the rendering of personal opinion, and it could be wrong. Of course the analyst believes in the correctness of the intervention when doing it, but opinions are subject to modification. Yet how does one eventually arrive at the best meaning for the patient? Primarily by experimentation, by discussions over time of different possibilities until patients reach points where they can say this works for me, and the analyst can agree. These points of agreement will have a relativity to them so that the degree of consensus will vary, but it is possible to reach an understanding about reservations to solutions that do exist and at the same time progress and even conclude the analysis. There is a general agreement that patients need to learn about themselves and put that learning to work so that they have better lives, while within that agreement there will be many views about how that learning best takes place, as well as what indeed are "better lives," and of course on the latter point, that will eventually be up to the patients based on their narcissism.

In addition to the separation-connection issue highlighting the role of narcissism, the controversy reflects the need for balance. In the separation emphasis the significance of the interpersonal field is neither sufficiently nor appropriately recognized, and autonomy is reactive to both instinctive demands and social-relational pressures to the point of constricting subjectivity. In connection theory the power of instinctual drives as subjective motivators is significantly diminished, and subjectivity is recognized within the context of relatedness, thus restricting autonomy. Both approaches attempt to redress the limitations of each other, and are reflective of the paradigm shifts noted by Rubin (1997) that are currently taking place, namely from drive to relations, and from positivism to perspectivism. As has been pointed out these are shifts in emphasis, and each categorization indicates broad trends without being able to capture the complexities or irregularities that occur. One of those complexities, from a personal point of view, remains appropriately addressing the development and the role of subjectivity, which is seen as still being subordinated, first to objectivism, and recently, to mutuality and intersubjectivity. There is an idealistic flavor to all this that is appealing, but skepticism remains as to its reality. Postmodern thinking could be employed here to dismiss the reality concept (Gergen, 1996), but Sampson (1993) has pointed out the reality is not in question, but interpretations of reality.

As a result, the interpretation of reality offered here represents a different slant than what is being offered either by separation or connection paradigms, or by past paradigms and paradigm shifts. The view in this chapter would move the emphasis to the distinctiveness and motivational power of subjectivity, rather than the forces that influence it. This is a trend that was initially reflected in giving power to the drives, but then mitigated by the ego and the superego so that the self becomes diminished as though it would not and could not adaptively self-control to relate to others. This trend reappears in the need for empathic responses from others, or recognition by others, but again is controlled by the need to empathize, to recognize the other as a subject as well as an object, with the implication, if not the overt declaration, that nurturing is an ideal that is a basic motivation that is impeded by reactive individuality. Both the separation and the connection model emphasize the goal of socialization, but for different reasons. In the separation model socialization is necessary for drive modification rather than being a primary goal itself. Thus although separation theory is criticized for leading to problems such as alienation and self-absorption, these are pathologies of individuality that reflect failures in adaptation, because the emphasis in separation theory is on self-control. In that regard various aspects of self-expression and creativity are limited by the theory, as are the satisfactions that can be derived from relationships. Connection theory attempts to make up for the emphasis on separation by attributing far greater motivational power to relationships, and uses the value of relationships to revise some other conceptions attached to separation theory, such as using male development as a norm (Gilligan, Rogers, & Tolman, 1991). However, connection theory further limits the potential of individuality and is unconvincing in regard to the basic motivational nature of socialization. Neither separation theory or connection theory adequately account for the power of narcissism, although their emphases make the point that self and social motivations both require major considerations in any model of human behavior. Building on the insights of both models as offering a different possibility is suggested, namely narcissism as the organizing principle of development, a view that is elaborated in the next chapter.

VIII
Narcissism As Organization

When Freud used narcissism as a psychoanalytic concept, he included what could be called the "good" and "bad" possibilities. This duality has not changed over time, appearing currently in healthy and pathological narcissism as different forms of self-interest. Narcissism includes both a state of subjectivity, that is a sense of being that is a self-representation, and a trait, the expression of subjectivity. Although narcissism has been used more often as a negative term than a positive one, it is not accurate to restrict its meaning to pathology. The richness, complexity, and totality of the concept of narcissism are best appreciated by defining narcissism as a personal perspective. The importance of understanding narcissism is emphasized by the increasing recognition and acceptance of subjectivity as a basic part of psychoanalysis (Markari, 1997).

Freud was struck by the idea that people are inevitably ambivalent. The recognition of the ongoing ambivalent self is noted by a number of contemporary theorists with different overall conceptual frameworks (Aron, 1996; Greenberg, 1991; Parker, 1995). Narcissism in all its diversity captures the disruptive vitality of our lives that involves the presence and resolution of conflict so that we can have *relatively consistent* feelings.

People are always motivated by what they consider to be their self-interest, their *personal perspective*, but there has been a reluctance to be this explicit about behavior being organized, and therefore motivated, in terms of narcissism because such a view appears to deny the importance of the needs of others and the concept of altruism. To state that everybody is motivated by what they believe is good for them, as individuals, appears narcissistic in a pejorative sense. However, such an appearance is deceptive and inaccurate. The satisfaction of the self is dependent on the satisfaction of others, but it is a false dichotomy to believe that one satisfies others at the expense of the self. Instead, it is necessary to realize that when this imbalance apparently occurs, it is because the person is factoring in a greater self-satisfaction by doing for others in that particular circumstance. The self-image or self-representation rests on how one wishes to perceive the self, which is intertwined with how others are likely to perceive the person. Thus altruism divorced from narcissism becomes an illusion. There are substitutions of goals for self satisfaction, in particular sublimation, but they are part of a narcissistic organization of the personality. This organization is fluid and includes behaviors that are indeed good for the self (healthy narcissism) and behaviors that are not good for the self (pathological narcissism). The latter originate nonetheless in the hope that they will be satisfying, but turn out not to be. The criteria for such satisfaction can be difficult to define and given the interactional nature of development, are generally reflective of others' reactions and social and ethical norms.

Thus there is little danger that operating from an organizing principle of self-interest is likely to result in the widespread exploitation of others. Healthy self-interest is a reflected appraisal that accounts for the interest of others, a point highlighted by the concept of intersubjectivity. However, there is the possibility of exploitation, whether of others or to the self, because intersubjectivity also illustrates the existence of separate selves in a dyad. Thus there are individual desires, and the potential for domination and submission. There is often a tension or dissonance between the wishes of the two subjects. Benjamin (1995a) has described this in terms of negating and affirming the other, the need to appreciate the other in order to relate affectively. In any relational process there will be a repetitive tension between mutuality and subordination. Greenberg (1991) points out that all relationships have their unsatisfactory aspects with inevitable frustrations. The way that relationships work, as well as other endeavors, are in terms of relative satisfactions and relative deprivations, with the self organized to attempt to limit the experiencing of deprivation. This is a modified pleasure principle in that it does not rest on the economics of energy distribution but on the experience of contextual pleasure which is individually variable.

Intersubjectivity is often depicted as gaining recognition in dialectic or dialogic tension wherein the subjects work out their differences in mutual discourse. In the therapy situation this tends to be primarily verbal discourse, but this is accomplished within the framework of separate narcissistic organizations. It is very useful to show the value of connections, and to illustrate the pitfalls of disconnections (Miller & Stiver, 1997), but there does not have to be significant opposition between self and others in conceptualizing motivation as narcissistic. A personal perspective by definition favors neither separation or connection, but the use of both in different ways at different times. To say that narcissism is the organizing principle of personality development is to make explicit what is going to be the meaning of subjectivity in any situation.

Motivation

The major motivations included in psychoanalytic theories tend to fall into either drive or relational categories. Such categorization does not involve full appreciation of either category, but it does stress the major emphases that color psychoanalytic thinking. These emphases have already been discussed in some detail in the preceding chapter on separation and connection. Within these categories there have indeed been a number of refinements. Greenberg (1991) has presented a critical review of the ways in which drive and relational concepts have been elaborated. It is apparent that motivational possibilities have been significantly expanded, although within all of the approaches there is at the same time a tendency to try for a restricted number of basic motivations. The result of such limitation is to have a categorically efficient model at the expense of specific refinements of motivation. Miller and Stiver (1997) take note of this problem when they designate their approach as relational, but point out that their "relational" model differs from others that neglect power differentials and cultural influences.

In considering the major motivational offerings all of them, libido, aggression, safety, competence, attachment, interaction, connection, etc., can be demonstrated as having significance. However, it seems that attempts to subordinate one or more to another are feasible only some of the time. The problem of attempting to in a sense discredit narcissism is that those who for example favor enhancing relationships may do so because it is their personal preference, not because people have a superordinate motive to be enhancing. Saying that does not diminish the value of relating, but it does make the point that it is a personal point of reference that causes preferences for mutuality or disengagement.

Thus another way to look at motivation is to notice that people are motivated to organize themselves. Significant components of such organization are found in sex, aggression, security, connection, etc., and the result is almost an infinite variety of motivational preference that are individualized. Thus, even if one disagrees with the specifics suggested by Pine (1990), he is right on target in proposing personal motivational hierarchies. Also of particular interest here is Schafer's (1983) observations that patients present personal narratives and analysts pursue certain storylines of development. Hermans and Hermans-Jansen (1995) depict people as motivated storytellers, with each individual having an ongoing personal narrative. They believe that these personal narratives are organized around two basic motives, self-enhancement and contact with others, a distinction akin to separation and connection. They make the point that these motives are not drives, but important goals with affective components involved in the personal construction of meaning, namely narcissism, although the authors do not call it that. Also, it is pertinent to add here that the influences of culture, gender, race and class are components of this narcissism, as Miller and Stiver (1997) point out so well. At the same time, it is the narcissistic perspective of these influences that represent the activity of motivation.

Another interesting feature of the self-narrative emphasis is the influence of affects which are considered to be the bridge between basic motives and the construction of meaning (Hermans & Hermans-Jansen, 1995). Consider the similarity of this reasoning to the view of Kernberg (1992) that affects are bridges between instincts and psychic drives. The organization of behavior and its expression are significantly influenced by affects, e.g., what feels good or bad. Thus one could consider that Freud did not have to go beyond the pleasure principle provided he accepted the paradoxes of pleasure.

Spezzano (1993) has presented a substantial exposition of the motivational influence of affects. He takes note of the many dualities that have been proposed as the basic motives, and suggests that rather than settle on one pair to which all human desires are reducible that one can accept the possibility of numerous predispositions, any one of which may dominate at a given moment in a given individual. He then makes the affective link by stating: "Each of these predispositions is subjectively experienced as a desire to maximize...or to minimize...a specific affect" (p. 152).

A democracy of affects is offered that is compatible with the democracy of desires, and affects are depicted in goal-directed terms, such as indicators of the state of the relational self, forms of communication, and predispositions to action. Affects at work are then illustrated by sexual excitement, the excitement of interest, feelings of certainty and perfection, and relational coordination. The motivational impact of affects is also illustrated in organizing developmental experience within intersubjective systems (Orange, Atwood, & Stolorow, 1997).

Motivation is most understandable as an organized system of needs/desires, feelings, and structure. The range of its components are broad, essentially limited by attempts at efficiency, but it is not necessary to accord superordinate status to drives, or relations, or specific affects, or particular modes of organization. It is true that certain wishes, feelings, and contexts have more frequency than others and thus are more likely to appear in patients' personal narratives or to be pursued as story lines by therapists. The work that has been accomplished in regards to highlighting the effect of anger, sexuality, separation, and connection is very helpful in understanding what are likely motivational forces, and the intertwining of bodily-based experiences with psychological representations is a key feature of motivation. Also, the contexts of motivation are frequently interpersonal but also can be "just personal," meaning self-referenced. The organized system is fundamentally personal and so it is narcissistic. If one tracks back any action to its source, that source will inevitably be the expectation of personal gratification.

The determination of what indeed will be self-pleasure is what I term the personal perspective, and it is reflective of a variety of outcomes that are considered personally desirable as well as being desired by others. Thus altruism has it apparent appearance, as does personal sacrifice, the good of others, and social, ethical, and moral values. There are of course people who are "bad," and all of us are open to that possibility in various ways, disconnections, exploitations, excesses, and distortions that can be considered pathological narcissism. Furthermore, the good-bad distinction is ultimately subjective and thus not fair, although attempts can certainly be made to make it equitable. Thus we have constructs such as justice and charity. However, people are motivated by their view of what is going to be personally gratifying rather than by perspectives that sound better, such as healing connections, or worse, as untamed desires. Narcissism is potentially adaptive through experience and potentially maladaptive in the same context. Our lives are in turn narcissistic mixtures.

In that regard the self is not reified or glorified as so separate from relational and cultural influences. Instead, consider the self as a construct or system that is temporal and spatial, impulsive and reflective, alone and together, ultimately organized in terms of subjectivity which in turn has been significantly shaped by objectivity (in the sense of the view of objects other than the self).

The understanding of motivation is developed in terms of a patient's personal narrative in the psychotherapy session. The following is a description of how that can occur. In this case the patient had been telling her therapist that she was starting to consider her behavior to be "passive-aggressive."

The patient said, "You know, the last session when I told you that when I was in the waiting room I told you I could hear you talking to someone else?"

"Yes."

"Well I know I told you that I felt you would want to know, that I was trying to be helpful, and you said that it was helpful to know that, and that you did not want anything that was being said to be overheard, but that you wondered if that was the only reason I was telling you."

"Yes, it also felt critical."

"It was, I felt I might be overheard, and that you should make sure I was not."

"Did you also believe I was unaware of the possibility, or even that I did not care?"

"I thought you cared, but that you didn't know. Well, maybe I thought you were being careless. (The patient laughs a little). I suppose that is saying you didn't care."

"I'm glad you told me so I can prevent it, but that day you were early, and the door had been left open by the previous person, and before I checked it I got a phone call and you overheard my portion of that call which wasn't, I don't know, particularly private, really one side of a conversation with a car service representative. In thinking about it I didn't mind if you heard it, but that doesn't change the fact that there was a lapse in privacy.

"I was angry about it. I mean, I wasn't just trying to be helpful."

"You were being critical?"

"Yes, and I don't like that image of myself. I mean, I realized I do it a lot, and I don't even seem to realize that part of it."

The patient then related other examples of providing "helpful" information. In all these instances the patient started with the premise that she was being helpful, but became aware that she was angry at the people, and sometimes also angry at their response to her attempts at assisting them.

The therapist said, "These scenes remind me of the situations between you and your mother where you feel criticized and she always tells you that she is just trying to be helpful."

"Yes, it is true. I act like her, and I don't want to be like her. I am angry, and it just comes out of me."

This segment illustrates the patient's personal perspective. She organizes her behavior in such a way that she can express her anger through apparent helpfulness, and she wants to be thought of as helpful, but she also wants people to do things the way she believes they should be done. She also has a desire to identify with her mother, and to be a mother in a controlling-helpful way, as well as to see herself as different from her mother. I am sure there are still other possibilities, so it is clear that multiplicities of motivations operate and are organized in accord with the patient's narcissism. In this case that precluded the view of herself as angry and replaced it with helpful until the therapy process revealed the mix. I believe it would be inaccurate to reduce her motivation to being passive-aggressive because she also intended to be helpful and was, but her personal perspective was restricted until she became aware of the hidden aspects of her motivation. The helpfulness was in service of her good image, which if she now wants to retain she will have to find a way to integrate her anger rather than keep it concealed from her awareness.

Development

A striking feature in current developmental theory is the evidence for the infant's early capacities for differentiation. I have suggested earlier that there is a rudimentary self from birth, and the self-concept, self-representations and object-representations, and relational patterns all develop more rapidly than had originally been conceptualized in psychoanalytic theory. This involves a reevaluation of the primacy of psychosexual and relational stages, but the idea of developmental phases remains of value as potential areas of success and failure, frustration and gratification, memory traces and sources of repetitive patterns. The limitations in predicting pathology or health in specific terms from developmental events, particularly from parenting styles, has been noted, but it is clear that parent-child interactions exert a significant influence on individual development. Certainly the importance of relational patterns has come to the fore and at the moment surpasses concerns with drive expression and gratification.

My focus is on the development of narcissism, particularly the growth of an adaptive personal perspective, namely one that works for the individual. This involves the integration of developmental experiences, and the understanding of pre-oedipal, oedipal, and post-oedipal relations and drive expressions are all useful here. The activity of narcissism can be illustrated in a contemporary proposal of the development of conflict (Greenberg, 1991).

Conflict is described in three contexts. The first is where the affects are described as "...pre-experiential and may have little or no connection with other people" (p. 137). The existence of this state requires notice because it supports the existence and persistence of the separate self as opposed to the idea that the self is always a relational construct. That view does not negate the importance of the child-caretaker context, or desires for connection, but argues for the coexistence and oscillation of separateness and connectedness. Both states are viable and have their attractions. The solitary state is both physical and affective, as well as illusory in a number of ways. Thus the infant develops within and connected to the mother, yet has a separate existence that involves the potentiality for greater separation. This separation occurs and increases in the developmental process, but at the same time the world of objects is expanded, dependency becomes interdependency, and fantasy is usually "peopled" by the presence of objects. Although the process of differentiation appears to be immediately present, it is also gradual, and thus the idea of "infant omnipotence" which is an illusion of independence. Of course the personal perspective at that point has to be inferred, and projective identification is a good example of such inferences. The guessing game continues in all developmental proposals, also with more support as verbalization and motility and affective sophistication all make their epigenetic appearances. What is important in regard to narcissism is the process of organization of the self in terms of intentionality. The existence of any person brings conflict and the need for resolution, so the person develops "life methods" to have a life, and this narcissism has to have a very early origin.

The second context for conflict is about an object, but preceding the relationship and being brought into the relationship, basically an expectation. In this setting it is more apparent to the person that separation and connection can threaten each other. Thus in being drawn to others, and in recognizing others, there is some comprehension of attending to the self. My impression is that the expectation is that one will get something from another, and that is included in the giving of something, whether it be a look, a smile, or a thing. The giving is to get a response, contact, acknowledgement, praise, even punishment, if desired in some way. Thus even the most optimistic connection theories (Miller & Stiver, 1997) do not provide a convincing case for a basic desire for intersubjectivity based on an early expectation of its value. One learns that this can be valuable, but again, it is self-referenced.

In seeking the contact, in trying to get, or to give to get, the third context appears, conflict with the object, and that is when intersubjectivity is particularly available to consciousness. The others are subjects as well, doing their own giving and getting in styles that are not perfectly conforming to the person seeking the interaction in the first place. The result of this growing awareness is the continued modification of one's personal views as to how to best satisfy the self. It is important here not to substitute how one would like people to be, or ideal ways of being, for people's real subjective states, which are more frequently ambivalent, mixed, and above all personalized. In this vein then, conflict keeps appearing and reappearing because it is an unending task to form and activate personal perspectives that provide sufficient self-satisfaction. In that regard, selfishness is both an obstacle and an aid, and the same can be said for existence of other people in one's life.

It is difficult for a person to even recall no less understand many developmental experiences, and all therapists are another step removed, so at best the patient's personal narratives are clues and point to directions. However, the value of conceptualizing the patient's life in terms of narcissism is that patients invariably do have views of their past that emphasize the "I". Patients tell you about themselves, and of course about others, but their view of it all is what the therapist gets and works with. In this context I think of Balint's idea that consciousness requires being a person, and that in turn requires an environment for projection. She saw the person as coming alive through imaginative perception, which goes beyond introjection and identification. There has to be a context, and I and someone else (Balint, 1993). At first I imagine that someone else to be parts of the self reflected by other parts, perhaps a core and its surround, with the latter growing with the differentiation of others. The self organizes imaginatively, and therefore fills in the memory blanks as well as coloring the present and creatively designing a future, all the time operating from a base of narcissism.

Although contextual theory is probably more of an attitude than a theory, it starts with the recognition of what I call narcissism. For example, "Intersubjectivity theory sees humans as organizers of experience, as subjects" (Orange, et al., 1997, p. 5). Although it moves on from there to insist that self-experience is based in relatedness to a point of exclusivity that bypasses a context of the facets of the self, or self-relatedness, it opens the way to intriguing understandings of developmental pathology. In this regard, delusions have often been viewed as the creation of a view that replaces an overly painful reality, a drastic form of self-defense. However, it is also possible to consider delusions as attempts to maintain a reality that is not too painful, but that is being withdrawn by others invalidating the feelings and perceptions of the individual (Stolorow, et al., 1987). In that sense the delusion is reality as the patient knows it, and reality is the delusion given the patient by the invalidating affective environment. There is an emphasis on what is missing in the experience, an absence of a continuous self, rather than what is present, a delusional self.

Another possibility appears in regard to shame. This feeling can be viewed as coming from the failure of a parent to support a child's pleasure in personal functioning. However, it is also possible to view shame as coming from malattunement by caretakers to painful or pleasurable affective states because of a need to develop a defensive ideal to counteract whatever the feelings are that are being invalidated. Dissociation is also looked at in a different light, not so much as a type of repression or even splitting, but as a type of self-organization that allows a separation from a painful environment and its replacement with a more tolerable environment. Whether one agrees with those different interpretations is not the issue, but that they have plausibility, and in particular, are framed in terms of self-organization, personal perspectives or what I call narcissism.

Contextual theory poses the possibility of making use of the various discoveries of psychoanalytic developmental theory, such as Freud's psychosexual stages, Mahler's stages of separation-individuation, and Klein's positions, to understand different moments of subjective experience in evocative and often metaphorical terms. These processes do not have to be considered universal, but can be decentered and fluid, and at times pointedly relevant. However, despite the assets of contextualism, all experiences do not arise out of relatedness and the individual's intrapsychic world is not only a part of an intersubjective system (Stolorow, 1997). This is a relational narcissism that describes only a part of the picture. Kohut (1971a) was more accurate when he stressed the internal construction of self-experience. This is not divorced form relational experience, but it is distinct, and it represents part of the origins of narcissism. Development is that there is an "I" and there is a "You", and there is interaction, interdependence, and separation, coexisting. An insistence on the relational person only, is just as problematic as a insistence on the isolated mind. There is considerable evidence that one frequently thinks in relational terms, and that intersubjectivity is an accurate description of significant ingredients of relating, but on does not always think in relational terms or even frequently conceptualize relations as being intersubjective.

Chodorow (1996) suggests the value of understanding development in terms of internal and external relations, the relations between inner and outer worlds, and meanings that are created internally as well as those that come from others or from the past. She notes that an infant invents an inner object world by providing self and objects with affects, drives, and feelings so that self and other are created. Her emphasis is on the influence of relations, but she also points out that infants create subjectivity. Development is being depicted in terms that leave room for a personal perspective, an "I" from birth. The interpersonal coexists, but it is necessary to keep emphasizing the psychobiological processes that feed an incipient self and that remain a part of the intersubjective self of later life.

Also of interest here are the comments regarding postmodernism by Elliott and Spezzano (1996). These include suggestion by various postmodern theorists in regard to the development of the self. One is that narcissism originates as a qualified representation of a self. Self-representations are incomplete, and unconscious dimensions are strikingly imaginary. In terms of developing a personal way of being, there is what is described as a "preliminary ordering of pre-self experience, otherness and difference" (p. 79). Elliott (1995) describes self-constitution as "rolling identification" (pp. 45-47).

By focusing on narcissism as the organizer of developmental experience it is possible to better understand the subjectivity of any patient's experience. Relationships are key factors in this subjectivity, but it is important to consider what personal gratifications are involved in relational matrices and intersubjective experiences. In that regard let me continue with the patient described earlier in the section on motivation.

The patient is describing her interest in having children, and she sounds particularly ambivalent. The therapist asks, "Do you feel you must have a child?"

"I suppose. How else would I be complete?"

"I don't know. What does being complete mean?"

"Well my mother had me, and my sister and brother. You know she was a mother."

"Yes, is that it, you want to be a mother?"

"It is part of growing up, like first you go to school, and you get a job, and you get married, and then you have a child."

"Well, you did everything up to the last part. How do you think it will feel, to have this child?"

"Scary, I suppose, but I don't want to think about that part yet, just the having."

"Next step, sort of, in being complete."

"Yes, and of course my husband wants me to do this."

"Is it part of being complete for him?"

"Yes, necessary, he's said it."

"So what he wants is part of it."

"Yes, and what my mother wants, I think. I'm not sure about that part."

"It would be a way to be like her."

"Sure, although I'm never sure about anything. I mean she wanted children, and I think my father didn't. I know they fought about that."

"Different ways to be complete."

"What do you mean? Wait, I think I can see it, for her it was children, for him it wasn't, or maybe it was me he didn't want."

"Do you remember feeling that, that he didn't want you?"

"No, well, I'm not so sure. He liked boys better than girls, but I think he probably wanted me. God, I'm not sure of anything. Maybe she didn't want me either. Maybe I was conceived because she thought she should have children, that's all, you know, nothing personal. Still, I remember how they fought, and sometimes I think I killed him. I mean, she had me, and maybe that did it, that killed him."

"You were born, he died."

"I know it wasn't that way in sequence, in time, because I was the oldest, but he did die."

"So if you have a baby, who will die?"

"Me, I suppose. I just want to go away from all this, not to have to decide, be by myself, never return, never have any part of it happening in the first place. Stupid idea I know. I have to face it, grow up."

"To be complete?"

"Yes, to be complete."

This segment of the therapy session illustrates the patient's perspective on her development, namely that she must do certain things, developmental tasks, to be a complete person, although it is not clear how that would make her happy in a "complete" sense. She also depicts an atmosphere of personal insecurity, of doubt about her parents' love for her, of a need to identify with both parents in different ways, to please her husband as part of being connected, but particularly to avoid it all. The desire expressed most often is to be "complete," but there is a strong pull to be alone as though completion might be possible that way, and at least for this session she remains ambivalent, struggling within herself about how to be "complete." Her personal perspective of her development is that there was something negative about her, an "incompleteness" that continues to be her lot in life, and that she is reluctant to alter, yet cannot rest with either.

Now in this segment there are a number of inferences that can be drawn around pre-oedipal and oedipal themes, as well as paranoid/schizoid and depressive positions, and certainly about mirroring and idealizing in regard to the cohesion of the self, given her stated desire to be "complete." The therapist has many directions that could have been pursued that were not at this point. Instead the focus was on elaborating developmental features connected to the completeness-baby connection. In that vein, her narcissism is illustrated as a very cautious approach to living her life that mixes separate space with connection in an unintegrated manner, and insists on guilt as well as inaction that both perpetuates the guilt of indecision as well as prevents the guilt of decision.

Subsequently she added a few statements that add to the picture of her narcissism. She said, "I cannot think of having something growing inside of me that will be taking from me," and she said, "I cannot live with the idea that I have produced nothing, that I have not completed what I should do." At some point she concluded, "If I get pregnant, well then, it will be decided, but perhaps I won't."

The therapist had asked, "What will be decided?"

"My life," she had said.

She got pregnant, but miscarried within a few months. Her life retained its destiny, she kept her personal perspective, she was not "complete." Although I have provided a limited amount of information about her development, and few inferences, I believe the material is sufficient to support the idea that she organized her life in such a way as to be incomplete, without specifying the details of such a state, but stressing indecision, ambivalence, guilt, avoidance, separation, and idealization in a restricted synthesis. Recognizing the personal perspective in terms of its possible motivations and its developmental antecedents, the next question is, how can psychoanalytic work proceed with this woman or any other individual's narcissism representing an organizing principle.

Treatment

A significant shift that has taken place in psychoanalytic treatment is the use of the therapist's subjectivity, or what I would call the narcissism of the analyst. This development is aptly described by McLaughlin (1996).

> First seeking to deny the existence of the analyst's influence, then attempting to eliminate it, we have only gradually come to acknowledge and cope with its being an inescapable component of the interplay of the dynamics of power between the analytic pair (p. 201).

Certainly the contextual approach of intersubjectivity advocates a way of working with the patient that highlights the subjectivity of both analyst and patient (Stolorow, 1997), an approach that is clearly reflected in the current works of Aron (1996), Miller and Stiver (1997), and Mitchell (1997). These authors stress a relational approach, but the theme is also reflected in other contemporary authors utilizing a different approach, such as a structural one. For example, both Gray (1986) and Busch (1995) disagree with the concept of the authoritarian, omniscient analyst and the submissive patient, and they take note of an increasing co-partnership between patient and analyst. Their emphasis is on encouraging self-reflection within an atmosphere of respect for the patient. Granted that these latter theorists are relatively dismissive of the curative power of empathic understanding, but they too have become more aware of the inevitable influence of the analyst's subjectivity. Thus Jacobs (1997) indicates that a prevalent view in psychoanalysis is that an analysis definitely involves the interaction of two people in terms of conscious and unconscious communications coming from both of these people, analyst as well as patient. Such a view reflects an ascendant recognition of the power of narcissism because it involves a focus on the subjectivity of interaction in the process of advocating an interactive model. This model can be compared with what is customarily considered the traditional model of interpretation creating insight which in turn leads to change. Of course it certainly involves an interacting dyad, particularly in the contemporary versions of the model (Bachant & Adler, 1997), but this structural approach is less interactive than a relational approach. The structural approach therefore attempts to be less subjective in its expression, although both approaches are well aware of the potential influence of the analyst's subjectivity.

Interaction itself is open to a variety of construction and expressions. These are traced by Mitchell (1997) in regard to both the Interpersonal and Kleinian traditions. Mitchell also describes different contemporary interactional methodologies, such as understanding the patient's conflicts through the stimulation of similar early developmental issues in the life of the analyst, or an engagement in regard to the current interpersonal states of the analyst and the patient, or the creation of combined subjectivity that involves projective identification and the analyst's internal objects. Mitchell indicates the potential utility of all three versions of interaction, which are drawn respectively from Jacobs (1991), Ehrenberg (1992), and Ogden (1994), but also points out "the entire manner in which the analyst participates with each patient is distinctly personal to that analyst...includes the analyst's very ideas of interaction and of psychoanalysis itself" (1997, p. 67).

Granted then that psychoanalysis is interactive and that the narcissism of both analyst and patient is involved, the questions are, what is the point of the interaction and how is narcissism used to make that point? There are going to be many answers to both questions, so let us look at a sample to clarify the general area of inquiry.

Busch (1996) offers the goals of analysis as increasing the patient's freedom of thought and the patient's ability to reflect upon the thoughts, namely the capacity for self-analysis. The process includes a significant relationship between analyst and patient in which trust and good intentions are major features, as is coparticipation. However, the major focus is on aiding the patient to change the way that the patient is thinking about personal conflicts. The interaction is focused on the analyst's concern with the patient's thoughts that includes "objectifying"

Narcissism and the Relational World

these thoughts as a way to foster the patient's self-reflections and thus at times being distant from the ongoing interaction. The central idea appears to be "stay with the patient's associations," so that the analyst is viewed as a participant guide. There is an assumption in this approach that the analyst's narcissism is either minimal or nonexistent in reflecting back to the patient what the analyst has heard. Busch describes the process as "representing the data" so that the patient can participate in developing insights, but he views this as a way of "objectifying" the data, and makes no comment about the subjectivity of representation by the analyst. He takes greater notice of this issue when the patient is less cooperative in providing associations, so that the analyst's subjectivity is the more apparent data, but his goal remains the same.

Bachant and Adler (1997) suggest that the work of the analyst is to facilitate the transference neurosis so that experienced repetitions can be transformed into recreations which in turn leads to greater understanding and improved personal integration. The analyst's tasks include listening, understanding, and maximizing the patient's self-expression in the session, which is contrasted with an emphasis on authenticity in the interaction. There is a strong belief in striving for neutrality that definitely acknowledges the influences of the analyst's subjectivity while putting the emphasis on the recognition of the patient's desires. Conceptualizing the analytic process in immediate interaction primarily is depreciated as ineffectively favoring current experience over primitive fantasy, reality, and psychic structure. In these illustrations of structural theory the patient's narcissism is detected in the organization of associations and the transference, but with an emphasis on what the patient is bringing to the analytic situation rather than patient-therapist interactions.

Using a model that emphasizes relational patterns, Mitchell (1997) considers the analyst's task to be a responsiveness that is self-reflective, being open to a multiplicity of intentions, listening to and following different levels of meaning, being guided by theoretical concepts as well as personal experience, and making clinical judgements about such crucial issues as when it is useful to talk about the patient-analyst interaction. The analyst's knowledge is reflected in the ability to understand the patient's experience in a way that is helpful, but that is one of many possible useful organizations. It is one analyst's best method, but not the best method, thus emphasizing the relative authority and knowledge of the analyst. Aron (1996) puts forth a similar position in indicating there is not the correct psychoanalytic method. He states that intervention is "on the basis of the analyst's own subjectivity...as it has been shaped in dialogue with the subjectivity of the other..." (p. 264).

Miller and Stiver (1997) consider their views to reflect a relational approach, which actually seems "especially" relational. The goal of therapy is mutual empowerment that involves understanding the origins and modes of disconnection and discerning ways to move to connection through a new relational experience between patient and therapist. Psychopathology is viewed as a number of different ways to try to stay unrelated and hide a basic desire for connection. In this model the therapist is expected to be open to her own feelings and to be willing to convey these feelings to the patient. This certainly emphasizes the subjectivity of the therapist, but it is designed to be intersubjectivity in which the therapist feels with the patient's experience and is moved by it. Self-disclosure is a likely part of this process. Aron (1996) has described self-disclosure in terms of both disadvantages and advantages, with the point being that neither anonymity or disclosure are designated hallmarks of effectiveness, and so either can be used and neither is out of the question. Ginot (1997) describes the use of reactive self-disclosure to help patients connect to disowned parts of themselves. What is being authenticated is the narcissistic organization of the analytic/therapeutic experience, although it is not being so categorized by the authors referenced.

Psychoanalytic practice has been increasingly influenced by the potential use of subjectivity. The traditional existence of the concept of countertransference makes it clear that there was always an awareness of the analyst's subjective states, but limited use was made of them. Now there is an ongoing interest in how to actively employ personal perspectives in the therapeutic process. This suggests the reactivation of narcissism as a very useful concept, and that it is helpful to think of the analytic procedure as being organized in terms of the narcissism of the people involved. Other organizing principles have viability, such as transference (Bachant & Adler, 1997) or mutual empowerment (Miller & Stiver, 1997), so the suggestions are not aimed at exclusivity, but more in terms of this too can be helpful, and it has an appeal in its complexity that has persisted throughout its history. It is in a sense a traditional psychoanalytic concept that is quite adaptable to numerous conceptualizations that at first seem singular.

Using the concept of narcissism as an organizer, it is helpful to begin the analytic process with the idea of trying to understand the patient's personal perspective, which can be conceptualized within structural or relational models but with an emphasis on hearing and processing and reflecting the patient's subjectivity. Of course this is carried out through the medium of the therapist's narcissism, the pathological aspects of which are modulated by the therapist's intention to be helpful to the patient. Thus mistakes are both possible and probable, but the therapist's gratification rests on whether or not the therapy is effective. In that sense the patient's needs are the therapist's needs, so that the therapist's narcissism increases his or her intersubjectivity, but that may not be the case for the patient. That is, the treatment process for the patient will be intersubjective in the sense that the patient will have an awareness of some personal aspects of the therapist, but its intersubjectivity for the patient will be restricted to the degree that the patient focuses on the therapist as an object rather than a subject. Such a happening is another aspect of the asymmetricality of mutuality in therapy which is also often altered during the course of treatment as the patient becomes more aware of objects as subjects.

I will illustrate the model of narcissism as a personal perspective by continuing with the case discussed earlier in this chapter. The focus in this segment is revealed in the session. The patient at this point has switched from talking about having a baby to discussing her struggles with her husband who is unhappy about his job situation.

She begins by stating, "I know this is not what we were talking about last session, but I'm having trouble with Jim (her husband) again."

"Oh?"

"He's unhappy about his job, as usual. I mean I can understand that he's under a lot of pressure, but I don't want him taking it out on me all the time."

"What do you want him to do?"

"I don't know, solve it, I suppose. I mean, he always does."

"Yes, he does, so what do you think he wants from you?"

"I know, I know, to be supportive. That is what he always wants, so much support. I mean, how much support does a person need?"

"How about you?"

"Sure, that's the problem. I need a lot of support from him, and he needs a lot of support from me, and how can I give him support, well I actually do, but there has to be a limit."

"He's gone over your limit."

"Over anybody's limit, but yes, over mine. I try, but it doesn't do any good."

"Is it possible that you stop at some point, maybe when you feel he should be feeling better but he doesn't seem to be?"

"Yes, I stop, and I get angry, and I tell him, get another job, and then he gets angry, and he yells at me, and I get more angry."

"Do you feel anything else?"

"Yes, afraid, afraid he will hurt me, not that he ever has, but he could."

"Do you think he wants to hurt you?"

"Probably not, but, you know, it reminds me of my parents, and my father did hit my mother."

"So you are afraid it will be the same, like your father and mother?"

"Well, I didn't want it to be that way. I mean, when I married Jim I was convinced he was nothing like my father, but he is turning out to be like him, with these rages."

"And you, are you turning out to be like your mother?"

"God, perhaps I am. My mother is so critical, and maybe that's what I am doing. What do you think, I mean I am trying to listen to him, but I get sick of it, and then I suppose I am critical."

"You asked me what I thought."

"Well, yes. I feel you must see me as critical, too."

"Too?"

"Along with Jim, with my mother, God everybody probably sees me that way, and I'm angry so much of the time. I don't like my life, or it's me I don't like."

The patient began to cry. The therapist was silent for a while. Then he said, "Let's put it together, sort of, you know, whatever it is that you don't like about you, and what you do like. Let's see where that takes us."

The patient organizes herself in this session by first explaining why she is choosing a particular topic. The therapist notices this and wonders what she would do if he said they should continue the theme of the previous session. So they start the session with the patient wanting to maintain herself by describing something that just happened, and the therapist having some desire to break up her system of immediacy, but deciding that is not the most helpful procedure. He also guesses that the "complete-incomplete" issue of past sessions will return. In essence it does, now in the form of her inability to both contain her husband and to have correctly discerned what it would be like to live with him. She was searching for safety from the danger of repeating the relationship of her parents, but now she feels as though that interaction has returned to haunt her. She is also again caught in the issue of differentiating herself from her mother, and is indecisive about her identity. Just for a moment she asks the therapist about his impression of her, and moves on from asking so quickly that he could have easily let it go, but he does not. However, she puts him in with others, and then moves from what others think about her to what she feels about herself. The therapist experiences her as both connected to him and disconnected from him. He wants to explore and to reassure, and he does both. He senses that she is struggling to find a place for herself, a psychic space that is not so haunted and conflicted, but trusts neither others or herself, so indecision, confusion, and anger are very prominent without a sense of comfort or hope being clearly articulated. Here is a narcissism of uncertainty that is reflected in the therapist's last comment, "let's see where that takes us."

Each of the analytic segments presented can be conceptualized in a variety of ways and the patient's verbalizations could be reacted to in ways other than described. My interest is to show that the concept of a personal perspective is present in motivation, development, and intervention, and that it provides a useful vantage point for understanding the patient. Narcissism is a categorical way of conceptualizing the patient, the therapist, and the analytic/therapeutic process that emphasizes the subjectivities involved. In particular it keeps the therapist focused on the question of what does the patient want, what do I want, how can we be together so that we both get what we want, and is the process effective. I believe that the therapist wants to be helpful to the patient, that the therapist's role is indeed so defined and in turn defines the healthy narcissism of the therapist. At the same time I am aware that all therapists have views on how best to be helpful at any given moment, and those views can and do differ from patient views, so getting together, the concept of mutual empowerment (Miller & Stiver, 1997) is very important for narcissistic satisfaction and will be played out dialectically (Aron, 1996). Also, it is necessary to both discern what a patient wants and to explore the consequences of getting it, as well as developing ways to expedite the desired changes. In my emphasis on the organizing power of narcissism I am featuring the necessity for the therapist to stay with the patient, e.g., "the analytic work must consistently remain focused on the patient's intentions" (Adler & Bachant, 1996, p. 1039).

Final Frame

At this point in the book I find myself facing what could be what Chused (1997) has depicted, in the context of analysis, as "informative experiences" (p. 1051). As she notes, a dissonance develops between realities that is disturbing, but the experience can be informative. Thus I note that in my experience people generally try to operate in their self-interest. At the same time, because self-interest or narcissism is an adaptive social construct in so many ways, the result is a relationally organized world with considerable interest in and respect for the feeling of others. This is not always the case of course, and then the result is pathological narcissism. The determination, specifically, of what is pathological and what is healthy can indeed be difficult. Such complexity creates a strong appeal for ideals and objectivity, but these may well be only approachable illusions that are temporary solutions to a vexing question of the moment. Nonetheless, such standards illustrate the value of trying to both have them and meet them. They help reconcile opposing subjectivities in the inevitable situations of everyone's life. Thus there is the relativity of objectivity, tinged as always by its interpreters, and the relativity of subjectivity, eternally pulled by the need for conflict resolutions. This is aptly depicted by Benjamin (1995a) as the breakdowns and restorations of the balance between the intrapsychic and the intersubjective in the process of learning to live with contradictions.

The therapeutic use of subjectivity can be enhanced by considering the motivational appeal of examining one's self states as a therapist responding to a patient. Whether it is an opening up of a line of personal thoughts and feelings, or a shutting down, the self-involvement is intriguing. There is a balance between attempting to listen only to the patient and getting lost in the self that analysts strive for and reach often enough. In so doing they use their own storylines and the patients' personal narratives in such a way that both patient and therapist stay involved, and awake.

Finally, analysts are being faced with some new narcissistic challenges. One of these is a growing patient population that is increasingly diverse culturally and ethnically, so that therapy is an unfamiliar situation requiring new attunements to patients' narcissism as well as to therapists' (Javier & Herron, 1998). Then, current mental health policy has fostered a new type of patient who presents with limited time and resources. Although I certainly advocate the development of health delivery systems that provide ideal environments for analytic practice (Herron, 1997), at the moment we have to live with the tension of finding ways to use psychoanalytic concepts and practices effectively with patients who afford us less than our previous average expectable environment. As a result, narcissism will continue to need to be revisited.

REFERENCES

Adler, E., & Bachant, J. L. (1996). Free association and analytic neutrality: The basic structure of the psychoanalytic situation. *Journal of the American Psychoanalytic Association, 44*, 1021-1046.

Adler, G. (1985). *Borderline psychopathology and its treatment.* New York: Jason Aronson.

Akhtar, S., & Anderson, J. A. (1982). Overview: Narcissistic personality disorder. *American Journal of Psychiatry, 139*, 12-20.

American Psychiatric Association. (1994). *Diagnostic and statistical manual of mental disorders.* 4th ed. Washington, D.C.: American Psychiatric Association.

Archer, J. (1996). Sex differences in social behavior. Are the social role and evolutionary explanations compatible? *American Psychologist, 51*, 909-917.

Aron, L. (1996). *A meeting of minds. Mutuality in psychoanalysis.* Hillsdale, NJ: Analytic Press.

Atkins, R. N. (1984). Transitive vitalization and its impact on father representation. *Contemporary Psychoanalysis, 20*, 663-676.

Atwood, G., & Stolorow, R. (1984). *Structures of subjectivity.* Hillsdale, N.J.: Analytic Press.

Auerbach, J. S. (1993). The origins of narcissism and narcissistic personality disorder: A theoretical and empirical reformulation. In J.M. Masling & R.F. Bornstein (Eds.), *Psychoanalytic perspectives on psychopathology.* (pp. 43-110). Washington, D.C.: American Psychological Association.

Bacal, H. (1990). Does an object relations theory exist in self psychology? *Psychoanalytic Inquiry, 10*, 197-220.

Bacal, N. A., & Newman, K. M. (1990). *Theories of object relations: Bridges to self psychology.* New York: Columbia University Press.

Bach, S. (1985). *Narcissistic states and the therapeutic process.* New York: Jason Aronson.

Bachant, J. L., & Adler, E. (1997). Transference: Co-constructed or brought to the interaction? *Journal of the American Psychoanalytic Association, 45,* 1097-1120.

Bachant, J. L., Lynch, A. A., & Richards, A. D. (1995a). Relational models in psychoanalytic theory. *Psychoanalytic Psychology, 12,* 71-81.

Bachant, J. L., Lynch, A.A., & Richards, A.D. (1995b). The evolution drive in contemporary psychoanalysis: A reply to Gill (1995). *Psychoanalytic Psychology, 12,* 565-573.

Badinter, E. (1981). *The myth of motherhood: An historical view of the maternal instinct.* London: Souvenir Press.

Bakan, D. (1966). *The duality of human existence.* Chicago: Rand McNally.

Balint, E. (1993). *Before I was I: Psychoanalysis and the imagination.* New York: Guilford Press.

Balint, M. J. (1968). *The basic fault.* London: Tavistock.

Becker, E. (1973). *The denial of death.* New York: Free Press.

Beebe, B., & Lachman, F. M. (1992). The contribution of mother-infant mutual influence to the origins of self- and object representations. In N.J. Skolnick & S.C. Warshaw (Eds.), *Relational perspectives in psychoanalysis* (pp.83-117). Hillsdale, N.J.: Analytic Press.

Bell Scott, P., Guy-Sheftall, B., Jones Royster, J., Sims-Wood, J., DeCosta-Willis, H., & Fultz, L. P. (Eds.). (1993). *Double stitch: Black women write about mothers and daughters.* New York: Harper.

Bem, S. L. (1993). *The lenses of gender.* New Haven, CT: Yale University Press.

Benjamin, J. (1988). *The bonds of love: Psychoanalysis, feminism, and the problem of domination.* New York: Pantheon.

Benjamin, J. (1991). Father and daughter: Identification with difference- a contribution to gender heterodoxy. *Psychoanalytic Dialogues, 1,* 277-299.

Benjamin, J (1992). Recognition and destruction. An outline of intersubjectivity. In N.J. Skolnick & S.C. Warshaw (Eds.), *Relational perspectives in psychoanalysis* (pp.43-60). Hillsdale, N.J.: Analytic Press.

Benjamin, J. (1995a). *Like subjects, love objects: Essays on recognition and sexual difference.* New Haven: Yale University Press.

Benjamin, J. (1995b). Sameness and difference: An "overinclusive" view of gender constitution. *Psychoanalytic Inquiry, 15,* 125-142.

Benjamin, L. S. (1996). *Interpersonal diagnosis and treatment of personality disorders.* New York: Guilford Press.

Bergman, S. J. (1995). Men's psychological development: A relational perspective. In R.F. Levant & W.S. Pollack (Eds.), *A new psychology of men* (pp.68-90). New York: Basic Books.

Bergmann, M. V. (1982). The female oedipus complex: Its antecedents and evolution. In D. Mendell (Ed.), *Early female development: Current psychoanalytic views* (pp. 175-202). New York: Spectrum.

Bergmann, M. V. (1987). *The anatomy of loving: The story of man's quest to know what love is.* New York: Columbia University Press.

Bernstein, I. (1983). Masochistic pathology and feminine development. *Journal of the American Psychoanalytic Association, 31,* 467-486.

Bibring, E. (1953). The mechanism of depression. In P. Greenacre (Ed.), *Affective disorders* (pp. 13-48). New York: International Universities Press.

Blanck, G., & Blanck, R. (1994). *Ego psychology. Theory and practice.* 2nd ed. New York: Columbia University Press.

Blatt, S. J. (1974). Levels of object representation in anaclitic and introjective depression. *The Psychoanalytic Study of the Child, 29,* 107-157.

Blatt, S. J., & Hermann, E. (1992). Parent-child interaction in the etiology of dependent and self-critical depression. *Clinical Psychology Review, 12,* 47-91.

Blatt, S. J., Quinlan, D. M., & Chevron, E. (1990). Empirical investigations of a psychoanalytic theory of depression. In J. Masling (Ed.), *Empirical studies of psychoanalytic theories,* Vol. 3 (pp. 89-147). Hillsdale, N. J.: Analytic Press.

Blechner, M. J. (1995). Societal prejudice, psychodiagnosis, and treatment aims. *The Round Robin, 11,* 9-12.

Blechner, M. J. (1996). Values, bigotry, and the aims of psychoanalysis. *The Round Robin, 11,* 7-9.

Bocknek, G., & Perona, F. (1994). Studies in self-representation beyond childhood. In J. Masling & R.F. Bornstein (Eds.), *Empirical perspectives on object relations theory* (pp.29-58). Washington, DC: American Psychological Association.

Bornstein, R. F. (1996). Beyond orality: Toward an object relations/interactionist reconceptualization of the etiology and dynamics of dependency. *Psychoanalytic Psychology, 13*, 177-203.

Bowlby, J. (1969). *Attachment.* New York: Basic Books.

Brennan, T. (1992). *The interpretation of the flesh: Freud and femininity.* New York: Routledge.

Brenner, C. (1991). A psychoanalytic perspective on depression. *Journal of the American Psychoanalytic Association, 39*, 25-43.

Brenner, C. (1993). Mind as conflict and compromise formation. *Journal of Clinical Psychoanalysis, 3*, 473-488.

Brenner, C. (1996). The nature of knowledge and the limits of authority in psychoanalysis. *Psychoanalytic Quarterly, 65*, 21-31.

Bromberg, P. M. (1983). The mirror and the mask: On narcissism and psychoanalytic growth. *Contemporary Psychoanalysis, 19*, 359-387.

Brooks, G. R., & Gilbert, L.A. (1995). Men in families: Old constraints, new possibilities. In R.F. Levant & W.S. Pollack (Eds.), *A new psychology of men* (pp.252-279). New York: Basic Books.

Brooks, G. R., & Silverstein, L.B. (1995). Understanding the dark side of masculinity: An interactive systems model. In R.F. Levant & W.S. Pollack (Eds.), *A new psychology of men* (pp.280-333). New York: Basic Books.

Burch, B. (1992). *On intimate terms: The psychology of difference in lesbian relationships.* Urbana: University of Illinois Press.

Burch, B. (1993). Heterosexuality, bisexuality, and lesbianism: Psychoanalytic views of women's sexual object choice. *Psychoanalytic Review, 80*, 83-100.

Busch, F. (1995). Beginning a psychoanalytic treatment: Establishing a psychoanalytic frame. *Journal of the American Psychoanalytic Association, 43*, 449-468.

Busch, F. (1996). The ego and its significance in analytic interventions. *Journal of the American Psychoanalytic Association, 44*, 1073-1099.

Butler, J. (1990). The pleasures of repetition. In R.A. Glick & S. Bone (Eds.), *Pleasure beyond the pleasure principle* (pp.259-275). New Haven: Yale University Press.

Campbell, A. (1993). *Men, women, and aggression.* New York: Basic Books.

Caplan, P., & Hall-McCorquodale, I. (1985). Mother-blaming in major clinical journals. *American Journal of Orthopsychiatry, 55*, 345-353.

Chasseguet-Smirgel, J. (1981). *Female sexuality.* London: Virago.

Chessick, R. D. (1997). [Review of the book Dynamic psychotherapy of the borderline patient]. *Psychoanalytic Psychology, 14*, 441-449.

Chodorow, N. J. (1989). *Feminism and psychoanalytic theory.* New Haven, CT: Yale University Press.

Chodorow, N. J. (1994). *Femininities, masculinities, sexualities: Freud and beyond.* London: Free Association Books.

Chodorow, N. J.(1996). Reflections on the authority of the past in psychoanalytic thinking. *Psychoanalytic Quarterly, 65*, 32-51.

Chused, J. F.(1996). The therapeutic action of psychoanalysis: Abstinence and informative experiences. *Journal of the American Psychoanalytic Association, 44*, 1047-1071.

Colarusso, C. A. (1990). The third individuation. The effect of biological parenthood on separation-individuation processes in adulthood. *The Psychoanalytic Study of the Child, 45*, 179-194.

Dahl, E.K. (1988). Fantasies and gender. *The Psychoanalytic Study of the Child, 43*, 351-365.

Dare, C., & Holder, A. (1981). Developmental aspects of the interaction between narcissism, self-esteem, and object relations. *International Journal of Psycho-Analysis, 62*, 323-337.

David, D.S., & Brannon, R. (1976). *The forty-nine percent majority: The male sex role.* Reading, MA: Addison-Wesley.

DeMarneffe, D. E. (1997). Bodies and words: A study of young children's genital and gender knowledge. *Gender and Psychoanalysis, 2*, 3-33.

Domenici, T., & Lesser, R. C. (Eds.) (1995). *Disorienting sexuality Psychoanalytic reappraisals of sexual identities.* New York: Routledge.

Eagle, M. N. (1984). *Recent development in psychoanalysis. A critical evaluation.* New York: McGraw-Hill.

Ehrenberg, D. (1992). *The intimate edge.* New York: Norton.

Eichenbaum, L., & Orbach, S. (1983). *Understanding women.* New York: Basic Books.

Elise, D. (1991). An analysis of gender differences in separation-individuation. *Psychoanalytic Study of the Child, 46*, 51-67.

Elise, D. (1997). Primary femininity, bisexuality, and the female ego ideal: A re-examination of female developmental theory. *Psychoanalytic Quarterly, 66,* 489-517.

Elliott, A. (1995). The affirmation of primary repression rethought: Reflections on the state of the self in its unconscious relational world. *American Imago, 52,* 55-79.

Elliot, A., & Spezzano, C. (1996). Psychoanalysis at its limits: Navigating the postmodern turn. *Psychoanalytic Quarterly, 65,* 52-83.

Erikson, E. (1968). *Identity: Youth and crisis.* New York: Norton.

Etchegoyen, R. H. (1991). "On narcissism: An introduction": Text and context. In J. Sandler, E.S. Person, & P. Fonagy (Eds.), *Freud's "On narcissism: An introduction,"* (pp.54-74). New Haven: Yale University Press.

Fairbairn, W. R. (1952). *An object-relations theory of the personality.* New York: Basic Books.

Fast, I. (1984). *Gender identity. A differentiation model.* Hillsdale, NJ: Analytic Press.

Fenichel, O. (1945). *The psychoanalytic theory of neurosis.* New York: Norton.

Fine, R. (1986). *Narcissism, the self, and society.* New York: Columbia University Press.

Finzi, S. V. (1996). *Mothering: Toward a new psychoanalytic construction.* New York: Guilford Press.

Fiscalini, J. (1993). Interpersonal relations and the problem of narcissism. In J. Fiscalini & A.L. Grey (Eds.), *Narcissism and the interpersonal self.* (pp. 53-87). New York: Columbia University Press.

Flax, J. (1990). *Thinking fragments: Psychoanalysis, feminism, and post modernism in the contemporary West.* Berkeley: University of California Press.

Fogel, G. I., Lane, F. M., & Liebert, R. S. (Eds.). (1986). *The psychology of men. New psychoanalytic perspectives.* New York: Basic Books.

Fonagy, P., Moran, G. S., & Target, M. (1993). Aggression and the psychological self. *International Journal of Psycho-Analysis, 74,* 471-485.

Formanek, R. (1982). On the origins of gender identity. In D. Mendell (Ed.), *Early female development: Current psychoanalytic views* (pp. 1-24). New York: Spectrum.

Fosshage, J. L. (1992). Self psychology: The self and its vicissitudes within a relational matrix. In N. J. Skolnick & S. C. Warshaw (Eds.) *Relational perspectives in psychoanalysis* (pp. 21-42). Hillsdale, NJ: Analytic Press.

Freedman, N. (1986). On depression: The paralysis, annihilation, and reconstruction of meaning. In J. Masling (Ed.), *Empirical studies of psychoanalytic theories*, Vol. 2 (pp. 107-150). Hillsdale, N. J.: Lawrence Erlbaum.

Freud, A. (1965). *Normality and pathology in childhood.* New York: International Universities Press.

Freud, S. (1905). Three essays on the theory of sexuality. *Standard Edition*, Vol. 7, pp. 125-145. London: Hogarth Press.

Freud, S. (1911). Formulations on the two principles of mental functioning. *Standard Edition.* Vol. 12, pp. 218-226. London: Hogarth Press.

Freud, S. (1913). Totem and taboo. *Standard Edition.* Vol. 13, pp. 1-161. London: Hogarth Press.

Freud, S. (1914). On narcissism. An introduction. *Standard Edition.* Vol. 14, pp. 73-102. London: Hogarth Press.

Freud, S. (1917). The taboo of virginity. *Standard Edition.* Vol. 11, pp.191-208. London: Hogarth Press.

Freud, S. (1923). The ego and the id. *Standard Edition.* Vol. 19, pp. 12-59. London: Hogarth Press.

Friedman, L. (1996). Overview: Knowledge and authority in the psychoanalytic relationship. *Psychoanalytic Quarterly, 65*, 254-265.

Friedman, L. (1997). Ferrum, ignus, and medicina: Return to the crucible. *Journal of the American Psychoanalytic Association, 45*, 21-36.

Friedman, R. (1986). The psychoanalytic model of male homosexuality: A historical and theoretical critique. *Psychoanalytic Review, 73*, 79-115.

Fromm, E. (1964). *The heart of man.* New York: Harper & Row.

Gabbard, G. O. (1990). *Psychodynamic psychiatry in clinical practice.* Washington, DC: American Psychiatric Press.

Gergen, K. (1994). Exploring postmodernism: Perils or potentials? *American Psychologist, 49*, 412-416.

Gilbert, L.A. (1988). *Sharing it all: The rewards and struggles of two-career families.* New York: Plenum.

Gilligan, C. (1982). *In a different voice.* Cambridge, MA: Howard University Press.

Gilligan, C., Rogers, A.G., & Tolman, D.L. (Eds.). (1991). *Women, girls, and psychotherapy.* New York: Haworth Press.

Ginot, E. (1997). The analyst's use of self, self-disclosure, and enhanced integration. *Psychoanalytic Psychology, 14,* 365-381.

Glover, L., & Mendell, D. (1982). A suggested developmental sequence for a preoedipal genital phase. In D. Mendell (Ed.), *Early female development: Current psychoanalytic views* (pp. 127-174). New York: Spectrum.

Goldstein, W. (1996). *Dynamic psychotherapy of the borderline patient.* Northvale, NJ: Jason Aronson.

Gottschalk, L. A. (1990). Origins and evaluation of narcissism through the life cycle. In R.A. Nemiroff & C.A. Colaruso (Eds.), *New dimensions in adult development* (pp.73-94). New York: Basic Books.

Gray, P. (1986). On helping analysands observe intrapsychic activity. In A. D. Richards & M. S. Willick (Eds.), *Psychoanalysis, the science of mental conflict: Essays in honor of Charles Brenner* (pp. 245-262). Hillsdale, NJ: Analytic Press.

Greenberg, J. (1991). *Oedipus and beyond: A clinical theory.* Cambridge, MA: Harvard University Press.

Greenson, R. (1968). Dis-identifying from mother: Its special importance for the boy. *International Journal of Psychoanalysis, 49,* 370-374.

Greenspan, S.I. (1990). A developmental approach to pleasure and sexuality. In R.A. Glick & S. Bone (Eds.), *Beyond the pleasure principle* (pp.38-54). New Haven: Yale University Press.

Grey, A. L. (1993a). A spectrum of psychoanalytic self theories. In J. Fiscalini & A.L. Grey (Eds.), *Narcissism and the interpersonal self* (pp.11-52). New York: Columbia University Press.

Grey, A. L. (1993b). The interpersonal self updated. In J. Fiscalini & A.L. Grey (Eds.), *Narcissism and the interpersonal self* (pp.145-175). New York: Columbia University Press.

Grinker, R. R., Werble, B., & Drye, R. C. (1968). *The borderline syndrome: A behavioral study of ego-functions.* New York: Basic Books.

Harris, J. (1995). Where is the child's environment? A group socialization theory of development. *Psychological Review, 102,* 458-489.

Hartmann, H. (1950a). Comments on the psychoanalytic theory of the ego. In *Essays on ego psychology* (pp. 113-141). New York: International Universities Press.

Hartmann, H. (1950b). Psychoanalysis and developmental psychology. In *Essays on ego psychology* (pp. 99-112). New York: International Universities Press.

Havens, L. (1993). The concept of narcissistic interactions. In J. Fiscalini & A. L. Grey (Eds.), *Narcissism and the interpersonal self* (pp.189-199). New York: Columbia University Press.

Herman, N. (1989). *Too long a child: The mother-daughter dyad.* London: Free Association Press.

Hermans, H. J., & Hermans-Jansen, E. (1995). *Self narratives: The construction of meaning in psychotherapy.* New York: Guilford Press.

Herron, W. G.(1995). Development of the ethnic unconscious. *Psychoanalytic Psychology, 12,* 521-532.

Herron, W. G. (1997). Restructuring managed mental health care. In R. M. Alperin & D. G. Phillips (Eds.), *The impact of managed care on the practice of psychotherapy* (pp. 217-233). New York: Brunner/Mazel.

Herron, W. G., & Herron, M. J. (1996). The complexity of sexuality. *Psychoanalytic Reports, 78,* 129-130.

Herron, W. G., & Javier, R. A. (1996). Some psychoanalytic conceptions about the genesis of poverty. *Psychoanalytic Review, 83,* 631-640.

Hofer, M.A. (1990). Early symbiotic processes: Hard evidence from a soft place. In R.A. Glick & S. Bone (Eds.), *Beyond the pleasure principle* (pp.55-78). New Haven: Yale University Press.

Hoffman, I. Z. (1983). The patient as interpreter of the analyst's experience. *Contemporary Psychoanalysis, 19,* 389-422.

Horney, K. (1933). The denial of the vagina. In H. Kelman (Ed.), *Feminine psychology* (pp. 147-161). New York: Norton.

Horney, K. (1950). *Neurosis and human growth.* New York: Norton.

Irigaray, L. (1985). *The sex which is not one.* Ithaca: Cornell University Press.

Irigaray, L. (1991). *The Irigaray reader.* Cambridge, MA: Blackwell.

Isay, R. A. (1986). Homosexuality in homosexual and heterosexual men: Some distinctions and implications for treatment. In G. I. Fogel, F. M. Lane, & R. S. Liebert (Eds.), *The psychology of men. New psychoanalytic perspectives* (pp.277-299). New York: Basic Books.

Isay, R. A. (1989). *Being homosexual.* New York: Farror, Strauss, Giroux.

Jacobs, T. J. (1991). *The use of the self.* New York: International Universities Press.

Jacobs, T. J. (1997). In search of the mind of analyst: A progress report. *Journal of the American Psychoanalytic Association, 45,* 1035-1059.

Jacobson, E. (1954). The self and the object world. *The Psychoanalytic Study of the Child, 9,* 75-127.

Jacobson, E. (1964). *The self and the object world.* New York: International Universities Press.

Javier, R. A., & Herron, W. G. (Eds.) (1998). *Personality development and psychotherapy in our diverse society: A source book.* Northvale, NJ: Jason Aronson.

Javier, R. A., Herron, W. G., & Yanos, P. T. (1995). Urban poverty, ethnicity, and personality development. *Journal of Social Distress and the Homeless, 4,* 219-233.

Joffe, W .G., & Sandler, J. (1967). Some conceptual problems involved in the consideration of disorders of narcissism. *Journal of Child Psychotherapy, 2,* 56-66.

Johnson, S .M. (1987). *Humanizing the narcissistic style.* New York: Norton.

Jordan, J. V. (1997a). A relational perspective for understanding women's development. In J.V. Jordan (Ed.), *Women's growth in diversity* (pp. 9-25). New York: Guilford Press.

Jordan, J. V. (1997b). Clarity in connection: Empathic knowing, desire, and sexuality. In J. V. Jordan (Ed.), *Women's growth in diversity* (pp. 50-73). New York: Guilford Press.

Jordan, J. V. (Ed.). (1997c). *Women's growth in diversity.* New York: Guilford Press.

Jordan, J.V., Kaplan, A.G., Miller, J.B., Stiver, I. P., & Surrey, J.L. (1991). *Women's growth in connection.* New York: Guilford Press.

Kaplan, A. G. (1997). How can a group of white, heterosexual, privileged women claim to speak of "women's" experience? In J. V. Jordan (Ed.), *Women's growth in diversity* (pp. 32-37). New York: Guilford Press.

Karon, B. P. (1989a). On the formation of delusions. *Psychoanalytic Psychology, 6,* 169-185.

Karon, B. P. (1989b). Psychotherapy versus medication for schizophrenia: Empirical considerations. In S. Fisher & R.P. Greenberg (Eds.), *The limits of biological treatments for psychological distress:*

Comparisons with psychotherapy and placebo (pp. 105-150). Hillsdale, N. J.: Lawrence Erlbaum.

Karon, B. P. (1992). The fear of understanding schizophrenia. *Psychoanalytic Psychology, 9,* 191-211.

Karon, B. P., & Teixeira, M. H. (1995). Psychoanalytic therapy of schizophrenia. In J.P. Barber & P. Crits-Christoph (Eds.), *Dynamic therapies for psychiatric disorders (Axis I)* (pp. 84-130). New York: Basic Books.

Karon, B. P., & VandenBos, G. R. (1981*). Psychotherapy of schizophrenics: The treatment of choice.* New York: Jason Aronson.

Karon, B. P., & Widener, A. J. (1994). Is there really a schizophrenic parent? *Psychoanalytic Psychology, 11,* 47-61.

Kernberg, O. F. (1975). *Borderline conditions and pathological narcissism.* New York: Jason Aronson.

Kernberg, O.F. (1976). *Object relations theory and clinical psychoanalysis.* New York: Jason Aronson.

Kernberg, O. F. (1984). *Severe personality disorders: Psychotherapeutic strategies.* New Haven: Yale University Press.

Kernberg, O. F. (1986). A conceptual model of male perversion. In G.I. Fogel, F.M. Lane, & R.S. Liebert (Eds.), *The psychology of men. New psychoanalytic perspectives* (pp.152-180). New York: Basic Books.

Kernberg, O. F. (1992). *Aggression in personality disorders and perversions.* New Haven, CT: Yale University Press.

Kernberg, O. F. (1996). The analyst's authority in the psychoanalytic situation. *Psychoanalytic Quarterly, 65,* 137-157.

Kernberg, O. F., Selzer, M. A., Koenigsberg, H. W., Carr, A. C., & Appelbaum, A. H. (1989). *Psychodynamic psychotherapy of borderline patients.* New York: Basic Books.

Kestenberg, J. S., Marcus, H., Sossin, K. M., & Stevenson, R., Jr. (1982/1994). The development of parental attitudes. In S.H. Cath, A.R. Gurwitt, & J.M. Ross (Eds.), *Father and child. Developmental and clinical perspectives* (pp.205-218). Hillsdale, NJ: Analytic Press.

Kimmel, M., & Messner, M. (1992). *Men's lives.* (2nd ed.) New York: Macmillan.

Klein, M. (1932). *The psychoanalysis of children.* London: Hogarth Press.

Klein, M. (1952). *Developments in psychoanalysis.* London: Hogarth Press.

Klein, M. (1980). *Envy and gratitude and other works.* London: Hogarth Press.

Klerman, G. L., Weissman, M. M., Rounsaville, B. J. & Chevron, E. S. (1984). *Interpersonal psychotherapy of depression.* New York: Basic Books.

Kohut, H. (1968). The psychoanalytic treatment of narcissistic personality disorder. *The Psychoanalytic Study of the Child, 23,* 86-113.

Kohut, H. (1971a). *The analysis of the self.* New York: International Universities Press.

Kohut, H. (1971b). Thoughts on narcissism and narcissistic rage. *The Psychoanalytic Study of the Child, 24,* 360-400.

Kohut, H. (1977). *The restoration of the self.* New York: International Universities Press.

Kohut, H. (1984). *How does analysis cure?* Chicago: University of Chicago Press. Kristeva, J. (1989). *Black sun: Depression and melancholia.* New York: Columbia University Press.

Kubie, L. (1974). The drive to become both sexes. *Psychoanalytic Quarterly, 43,* 344-426.

Lamb, M. E. (1977). The development of parental preferences in the first two years of life. *Sex Roles, 3,* 475-497.

Lansky, M. R. (1989). The parental imago. In S.H. Cath, A.R. Gurwitt, & J.M. Ross (Eds.), *Father and child. Developmental and clinical perspectives* (pp.27-45). Hillsdale, NJ: Analytic Press.

Lansky, M. R. (1992). *Fathers who fail. Shame and psychopathology in the family system.* Hillsdale, NJ: Analytic Press.

Lasky, R (1993). *Dynamics of development and the therapeutic process.* Northvale, NJ: Jason Aronson.

Lazur, R. F., & Majors, R. (1995). Men of color: Ethnocultural variations of male gender role strain. In R.F. Levant & W.S. Pollack (Eds.), *A new psychology of men* (pp.337-358). New York: Basic Books.

Lee, R. P., & Martin, J.C. (1991). *Psychotherapy after Kohut. A textbook of self psychology.* Hillsdale, NJ: Analytic Press.

Lerner, H. G. (1991). *Women in therapy.* Northvale, NJ: Jason Aronson.

Levant, R. F. (1995). Toward the reconstruction of masculinity. In R.F. Levant & W.S. Pollack (Eds.), *A new psychology of men* (pp.229-251). New York: Basic Books.

Levant, R. F. (1996). The new psychology of men. *Professional Psychology: Research and Practice, 27,* 259-265.

Levant, R. F., & Pollack, W.S. (Eds.). (1995). *A new psychology of men*. New York: Basic Books.

Lewes, K. (1995). *Psychoanalysis and male homosexuality*. Northvale, NJ: Jason Aronson.

Lichtenberg, J .D. (1983). *Psychoanalysis and infant research*. Hillsdale, NJ: Analytic Press.

Lichtenberg, J. D. (1989). *Psychoanalysis and motivation*. Hillsdale, NJ: Analytic Press.

Lichtenberg, J. D. (1991). What is a selfobject? *Psychoanalytic Dialogues, 1,* 455-479.

Lichtenberg, J. D., Lachmann, F. M., & Fosshage, J. L. (1992). *Self and motivational systems. Toward a theory of psychoanalytic technique*. Hillsdale, NJ: Analytic Press.

Luborsky, L., Mark, D., Hale, A. V., Papp, C., Goldsmith, B., & Cacciola, J. (1995). Supportive-expressive dynamic psychotherapy of depression: A time-limited version. In J. P. Barber & P. Crits-Cristoph (Eds.), *Dynamic therapies for psychiatric disorders (Axis I)* (pp. 13-42). New York: Basic Books.

Mahler, M.S. (1968). *On human symbiosis and the vicissitudes of individuation*. New York: International Universities Press.

Mahler, M. S., Pine, F., & Bergman, A. (1975). *The psychological birth of the human infant*. New York: Basic Books.

Majors, R., & Billson, J.M. (1992). *Cool pose: The dilemma of black manhood in America*. New York: Lexington Books.

Markari, G. J. (1997). Current conceptions of neutrality and abstinence. *Journal of the American Psychoanalytic Association, 45,* 1231-1239.

Mayer, E. L. (1995). The phallic castration complex and primary femininity: Paired developmental lines toward female gender identity. *Journal of the American Psychoanalytic Association, 43,* 17-38.

McLaughlin, J. T. (1996). Power, authority, and influence in the analytic dyad. *Psychoanalytic Quarterly, 65,* 201-235.

McWilliams, N. (1994). *Psychoanalytic diagnosis*. New York: Guilford Press.

Meissner, W. W. (1984). *The borderline spectrum*. New York: Jason Aronson.

Meissner, W. W. (1988). *Treatment of patients in the borderline spectrum*. Northvale, NJ: Jason Aronson.

Merchant, C. (1980). *The death of nature: Women, ecology, and the scientific revolution.* New York: Harper & Ross.

Miller, A. (1979). Depression and grandiosity as related forms of narcissistic disturbances. *International Journal of Psycho-Analysis, 6,* 61-76.

Miller, J. B. (Ed.). (1973). *Psychoanalysis and women.* New York: Brunner/Mazel.

Miller, J. B., & Stiver, I. P. (1997). *The healing connection: How women form relationships in therapy and in life.* Boston: Beacon Press.

Mirande, A. (1985). *The Chicano experience.* Notre Dame, IN: University of Notre Dame Press.

Mitchell, J. (1974). *Psychoanalysis and feminism.* New York: Penguin

Mitchell, S. A. (1988). *Relational concept in psychoanalysis. An integration.* Cambridge, MA: Harvard University Press.

Mitchell, S. A. (1992). True selves, false selves, and the ambiguity of authenticity. In N.J. Skolnick & S.C. Warshaw (Eds.), *Relational perspectives in psychoanalysis* (pp.1-20). Hillsdale, NJ: Psychoanalytic Press.

Mitchell, S. A. (1993). *Hope and dread in psychoanalysis.* New York: Basic Books.

Mitchell, S. A. (1997). *Influence and autonomy in psychoanalysis.* Hillsdale, NJ: Analytic Press.

Modell, A.H. (1968). *Object love and reality.* New York: International Universities Press.

Modell, A. H. (1994). Common ground or divided ground. *Psychoanalytic Inquiry, 14,* 201-211.

Montrelay, M. (1993). Inquiry into femininity. In D. Brien (Ed.), *The gender conundrum: Contemporary perspectives of femininity and masculinity.* New York: Routledge.

Moore, B. E. (1975). Toward a clarification of the concept of narcissism. *The Psychoanalytic Study of the Child, 30,* 243-276.

Morgan, A. C. (1997). Application of infant research to psychoanalytic theory and therapy. *Psychoanalytic Psychology, 14,* 315-336.

Morrison, A. P. (1986). Introduction. In A. P. Morrison (Ed.), *Essential papers on narcissism* (pp. 1-10). New York: New York University Press.

Muir, R.C. (1989). Fatherhood from the perspective of object relations theory and relational systems theory. In S.H. Cath, A.R. Gurwitt, & J.M. Ross (Eds.), *Father and child. Developmental and clinical perspectives* (pp.47-61). Hillside, NJ: Analytic Press.

Murray, J.M. (1964). Narcissism and the ego ideal. *Journal of the American Psychoanalytic Association, 12,* 477-511.

Neubauer, P.B. (1986). Reciprocal effects of fathering on parent and child. In G.I. Fogel, F.M. Lane, & R.S. Liebert (Eds.), *The psychology of men. New psychoanalytic perspectives* (pp.213-228). New York: Basic Books.

Oakley, A. (1980). *Women confined: Towards a sociology of childbirth.* Oxford: Martin Robertson.

Ogden, T. (1994). *Subjects of analysis.* Northdale, NJ: Aronson.

Orange, D. M., Atwood, G. E., & Stolorow, R. D. (1997). *Working intersubjectively: Contextualism in psychoanalytic practice.* Hillsdale, NJ: Analytic Press.

Ornstein, P. H. (1991). From narcissism to ego psychology to self psychology. In J. Sandler, E.S. Person, and P. Fonagy (Eds.), *Freud's "On narcissism: An introduction* (pp. 175-194). New Haven: Yale University Press.

Parker, R. (1995). *Mother love/mother hate: The power of maternal ambivalence.* New York: Basic Books.

Patterson, C. (1992). Children of lesbian and gay parents. *Child Development, 63,* 1025-1042.

Phoenix, A., Woollett, A., & Lloyd, E. (Eds.). (1991). *Motherhood: Meanings, practices, and ideologies.* Newbury Park, CA: Sage.

Piaget, J., & Inhelder, B. (1959). *The psychology of the child.* New York: Basic Books.

Pine, F. (1990). *Drive, ego, object, and self. A synthesis for clinical work.* New York: Basic Books.

Pleck, J. H. (1981). *The myth of masculinity.* Cambridge, MA: MIT Press.

Pleck, J. H. (1987). American fathering in historical perspective. In M.S. Kimmel (Ed.), *Changing men: New directions in research on men and masculinity* (pp.83-97). Beverly Hills, CA: Sage.

Pleck, J. H. (1995). The gender role strain paradigm: An update. In R.F. Levant & W.S. Pollack (Eds.), *A new psychology of men* (pp.11-32). New York: Basic Books.

Pollack, W. S. (1995). No man is an island: Toward a new psychoanalytic psychology of men. In R.F. Levant & W.S. Pollack (Eds.), *A new psychology of men* (pp.33-67). New York: Basic Books.

Pruett, K. D. (1983). Infants of primary nurturing fathers. *The Psychoanalytic Study of the Child, 38,* 257-277.

Pruett, K. D., & Litzenberger, B. (1992). Latency development in children of primary nurturing fathers. *The Psychoanalytic Study of the Child, 47,* 85-101.

Pulver, S. E. (1970). Narcissism. The term and the concept. *Journal of the American Psychoanalytic Association, 18,* 319-341.

Rank, O. (1945). *Will therapy and truth and reality.* New York: Knopf.

Raphael-Leff, J. (1991). *Psychological processes of childbearing.* New York: Chapman and Hall.

Raphael-Leff, J. (1993). *Pregnancy: The inside story.* London: Sheldon Press.

Receiving line. (December 24, 1995). *The New York Times Magazine,* p.8.

Reich, A. (1953). Narcissistic object choice in women. *Journal of the American Psychoanalytic Association, 1,* 22-44.

Reich, A. (1960). Pathological forms of self-esteem regulation. *The Psychoanalytic Study of the Child, 15,* 215-232.

Renik, O. (1990). Comments on the clinical analysis of anxiety and depressive affect. *Psychoanalytic Quarterly, 59,* 226-248.

Renik, O. (1993). Analytic interaction: Conceptualizing technique in light of the analyst's irreducible subjectivity. *Psychoanalytic Quarterly, 62,* 553-571.

Renik, O. (1996). The perils of neutrality. *Psychoanalytic Quarterly, 65,* 445-517.

Riophe, H., & Galenson, E. (1981). *Infantile origins of sexual identity.* New York: International Universities Press.

Rosenman, S. (1981). Narcissus of the myth: An essay on narcissism and victimization. In S. Tuttman, C. Kaye, & M. Zimmerman (Eds.), *Object and self: A developmental approach* (pp.527-548). New York: International Universities Press.

Ross, J. M. (1982/1994). In search of fathering: A review. In S.H. Cath, A.R. Gurwitt, & J.M. Ross (Eds.), *Father and child. Developmental and clinical perspectives* (pp.21-32). Hillside, NJ: Analytic Press.

Rothstein, A. (1979). An exploration of the diagnostic term "narcissistic personality disorder." *Journal of the American Psychoanalytic Association, 27,* 893-912.

Rothstein, A. (1984). *The narcissistic pursuit of perfection.* New York: International Universities Press.

Rothstein, A. (1986). The theory of narcissism: An object-relations perspective. In A. P. Morrison (Ed.), *Essential papers on narcissism* (pp. 308-320). New York: New York University Press.

Rotundo, E.A. (1987). Patriarchs and participants: A historical perspective on fatherhood in the United States. In M. Kaufman (Ed.), *Beyond patriarchy: Essays by men on pleasure, power, and change* (pp.64-80). Toronto: Oxford University Press.

Rotundo, E.A. (1993). *American manhood. Transformations in masculinity from the revolution to the modern era.* New York: Basic Books.

Rubin, S. S. (1997). Self and object in the postmodern world. *Psychotherapy, 34,* 1-10.

Sampson, E. E. (1993). Identity politics: Challenges to psychology's understanding. *American Psychologist, 48,* 1219-1230.

Samuels, A. (1989). *The plural psyche: Personality, morality and the father.* New York: Routledge.

Samuels, A. (1993). *The political psyche.* New York: Routledge.

Sandler, J. (1986). Comments on the self and its objects. In R.L. Lax, S. Bach, & R. J. Burland (Eds.), *Self and object constancy* (pp.96-107). New York: Guilford Press.

Sandler, J., Person, E. S., & Fonagy, P. (Eds.). (1991). *Freud's "On narcissism: An introduction."* New Haven: Yale University Press.

Schafer, R. (1968). *Aspects of internalization.* New York: International Universities Press.

Schafer, R. (1983). *The analytic attitude.* New York: Basic Books.

Schwaber, E. A. (1992). Countertransference: The analyst's retreat from the patient's vantage point. *International Journal of Psychoanalysis, 73,* 349-362.

Shane, M., & Shane, E. (1980). Psychoanalytic developmental theories of the self: An integration. In A. Goldberg (Ed.), *Advances in self psychology* (pp.23-46). New York: International Universities Press.

Spezzano, C. (1993). *Affect in psychoanalysis: A clinical synthesis.* Hillsdale, NJ: The Analytic Press.

Spiegel, L. A. (1959). The self, the sense of self, and perception. *The Psychoanalytic Study of the Child, 14,* 81-109.

Spitz, R. A. (1959). *A genetic field theory of ego formation. Its implications for pathology.* New York: International Universities Press.

Spitz, R. A. (1965). *The first year of life.* New York: International Universities Press.

Spotnitz, H., & Resnikoff, P. (1954). The myth of narcissus. *Psychoanalytic Review, 41,* 173-181.

Stern, D. N. (1985). *The interpersonal world of the infant: A review from psychoanalysis and developmental psychology.* New York: Basic Books.

Stoller, R. J. (1977). Primary femininity. In H. P. Blum (Ed.), *Female psychology: Contemporary psychoanalytic views* (pp. 59-78). New York: International Universities Press.

Stoller, R. J. (1985). *Presentations of gender.* New Haven: Yale University Press.

Stolorow, R. D. (1975). Toward a fundamental definition of narcissism. *International Journal of Psycho-Analysis, 56,* 179-185.

Stolorow, R. D. (1997). Dynamic, dyadic, intersubjective systems: An evolving paradigm for psychoanalysis. *Psychoanalytic Psychology, 14,* 337-346.

Stolorow, R. D., & Atwood, G. E. (1992). *Contexts of being. The intersubjective foundations of psychological life.* Hillsdale, N.J.: Analytic Press.

Stolorow, R., Brandchaft, B., & Atwood, G. (1987). *Psychoanalytic treatment: An intersubjective approach.* Hillsdale, NJ: Analytic Press.

Sugarman, A. (1995). Psychoanalysis: Treatment of conflict or deficit? *Psychoanalytic Psychology, 12,* 55-70.

Sugarman, A., & Wilson, A. (1995). Introduction to the section: Contemporary structural analysts critique relational theories. *Psychoanalytic Psychology, 12,* 1-8.

Sullivan, H. S. (1940). *Conceptions of modern psychiatry.* New York: Norton.

Sullivan, H. S. (1954). *The psychiatric interview.* New York: Norton.

Suttie, I. D. (1935). *The origins of love and hate.* London: Kegan Paul.

Tabin, J. K. (1995). Notes on homosexuality. *The Round Robin, 11,* 1-6.

Tabin, J. K. (1996). Homosexuality: Part II. *The Round Robin, 11,* 1-6.

Teicholtz, J. G. (1978). A selective review of the psychoanalytic literature on theoretical conceptualizations of narcissism. *Journal of the American Psychoanalytic Association, 26,* 831-862.

Tubert, S. (1997). Deconstructing maternal desire. *Free Associations, 38,* 235-257.

Tyson, P. (1982/1994). The role of the father in gender identity, urethral erotism, and phallic narcissism. In S.H. Cath, A.R. Gurwitt, & J.M. Ross (Eds.), *Father and child. Developmental and clinical perspectives* (pp.175-188). Hillside, NJ: Analytic Press.

Tyson, P. (1994). Bedrock and beyond: An examination of the clinical utility of contemporary theories of female psychology. *Journal of the American Psychoanalytic Association, 42,* 447-468.

Tyson, P., & Tyson, R. L. (1990). *Psychoanalytic theories of development: An integration.* New Haven: Yale University Press.

Vans Mens-Verhulst, J., Schreurs, K., & Woertman, L. (Eds.). (1994). *Daughtering and mothering: female subjectivity reanalyzed.* New York: Routledge.

Volkan, V. (1986). The narcissism of minor differences in the psychological gap between nations. *Psychoanalytic Inquiry, 6,* 175-191.

Walkerdine, V., & Urwin, C. (1985). *Language, gender and childhood.* London: Routledge.

Welldon, E.V. (1988). *Mother, madonna, whore: The idealization and denigration of motherhood.* London: Free Association Books.

Welt, S.R., & Herron, W.G. (1990). *Narcissism and the psychotherapist.* New York: Guilford Press.

Werman, D.S. (1988). Freud's "narcissism of minor differences": A review and reassessment. *Journal of the American Academy of Psychoanalysis, 16,* 451-459.

Westen, D. (1990). The relations among narcissism, egocentrism, self-concept, and self-esteem: Experimental, clinical, and theoretical considerations. *Psychoanalysis and Contemporary Thought, 13,* 183-239.

Wink, P. (1991). Two faces of narcissism. *Journal of Personality and Social Psychology, 61,* 590-597.

Winnicott, D.W. (1958). *Collected papers: Through paediatrics to psychoanalysis.* New York: Basic Books.

Winnicott, D.W. (1965). *The maturational processes and the facilitating environment: Studies in the theory of emotional development.* Madison, CT: International Universities Press.

Wolf, E.S. (1980). On the developmental lines of selfobject relations. In A. Goldberg (Ed.), *Advances in self psychology* (pp.117-130). New York: International Universities Press.

INDEX

272 Narcissism and the Relational World

226, 266
Resnikoff, P., 2, 267
Richarsds, A., 204, 252, 257
Riophe, H., 36, 266
Rogers, A., 227, 257
Rosenman, S., 2, 267
Ross, J., 69, 261, 262, 264,
267, 269
Rothstein, A., 15, 19, 125,
267
Rotundo, E., 68, 69, 267
Rounsiville, B., 141, 262
Rubin, S., 227, 267
Sampson, E., 228, 267
Samuels, A., 112, 267
Sandler, J., 4, 5, 6, 28, 256,
265, 267
Schafer, R., 7, 233, 267
Schizophrenia, 128-141
Schreuss, K., 122
Schwaber, E., 182, 267
Self, 4, 5, 7, 25
  core, 34
  definition, 26-29, 36
  depreciating, 122
  development, 90
  endogenous, 26
  esteem, 6, 9
  experience, 7, 27, 50
  feminine, 118
  idealization, 6
  interactional, 26
  interest, 5, 7
  loss, 152, 153
  perspective, 48,
  psychology, 12, 13, 220
  representation, 4, 26, 28,
  202
  satisfaction, 230
  selfobject, 220

sense, 34, 36
separate, 218
structure, 7
system, 26-27, 234
Selzer, M., 153, 261
Separation, 33, 34, 36, 58,
201-207, 217, 225, 227, 228
Separation-individuation, 207
Sexual desire, 120
Shane, E., 29, 267
Shane, M., 29, 267
Sims-Wood, J., 252
Silverstein, L., 52, 57, 61, 70,
254
Skolnick, N., 252, 264
Socialization, 215
Sossin, K., 59, 261
Speigel, L., 5, 267
Spezzano, C., 224, 233, 239,
256, 267
Spitz, R., 7, 34, 267
Spotnitz, H., 2, 267
Stern, D., 17, 33-36, 38, 268
Stevenson, R., 59, 261
Stiver, I., 53, 232-233, 237,
243, 245, 248, 261, 264
Stoller, R., 40, 102, 268
Stolorow, 7, 9, 10, 12, 21,
26, 220, 233, 238, 264, 268
Structural theory, 201, 204-
206, 243
Subjectivity, 203, 225, 228,
245
Sublimation, 229
Submission, 230
Sugarman, A., 204, 168
Sullivan, H., 15, 26, 268
Surrey, J., 53, 261
Suttie, I., 14, 268
Superego, 35, 67, 206

About the Author

William G. Herron, Ph.D., A.B.P.P., is Professor, Department of Psychology, St. John's University, Jamaica, NY. He is a faculty member, Senior supervisor, and training analyst at the Contemporary Center for Advanced Psychoanalytic Studies in Livingston, NJ. Co-author of *Narcissism and the Psychotherapist* and *Money Matters: The Fee in Psychotherapy and Psychoanalysis*, and co-editor of *Domestic Violence: Assessment and Treatment* and *Personality Development and Psychotherapy in Our Diverse Society*, Dr. Herron is in private practice in Woodcliff Lake, NJ.